The
CMS
Survey
Coordinator's
Handbook

Jeffrey T. Coleman

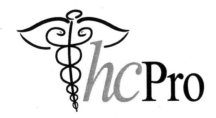

Jeffrey T. Coleman, Author
Jay Kumar, Editor
Brian Driscoll, Executive Editor
John Novack, Group Publisher
Susan Darbyshire, Cover Designer
Jackie Diehl Singer, Graphic Artist

Liza Banks, Proofreader
Darren Kelly, Books Production Supervisor
Paul Singer, Layout Artist
Susan Darbyshire, Art Director
Claire Cloutier, Production Manager
Jean St. Pierre, Director of Operations

Advice given is general. Readers should consult professional counsel for specific legal, ethical, or clinical questions.

Arrangements can be made for quantity discounts. For more information, contact:

HCPro, Inc.
P.O. Box 1168
Marblehead, MA 01945
Telephone: 800/650-6787 or 781/639-1872
Fax: 781/639-2982
E-mail: *customerservice@hcpro.com*

Visit HCPro at its World Wide Web sites:
www.hcpro.com and *www.hcmarketplace.com*

Table of contents

About the author

Jeffrey T. Coleman

Jeffrey T. Coleman worked for the New York state Department of Health as a surveyor for 28 years, retiring in 2004. He was assistant program director for hospital and primary care services in the western region of New York, covering 17 counties. He was responsible for the eight-county Buffalo office, establishing and running federal and state surveys in all types of facilities, including 31 hospitals. Coleman also assumed oversight and survey responsibilities for 60 diagnostic and treatment centers, which include ambulatory surgery centers, primary care clinics, renal dialysis centers, speech and hearing centers, and eight local health departments.

Introduction

Accrediting organizations, including the federal government, have come under continuing pressure to ensure some form of ongoing oversight of healthcare organizations. In the recent past, negative media reports, complaints from patients, and increased scrutiny of Centers for Medicare & Medicaid Services (CMS) oversight of the surveillance process have increased the probability that sooner or later your healthcare facility will be monitored by CMS.

This book is intended for the person or persons in the facility who will be the primary point of contact for the CMS surveyor(s), and the one most responsible for ensuring that the survey gets completed. But how does the coordinator control what the CMS surveyors do?

The answer lies in a number of steps that are taken before any survey begins, and which are carried through until the survey is considered closed by CMS.

This involves not only preparation on an ongoing basis, but also effective management of time, resources, and staff while the survey is underway. Last, it involves keen listening skills, knowledge of what surveyors are after, and an ability to express corrective action in a positive, not defensive, format.

This guide also provides the survey coordinator guidance for specific Conditions of Participation (CoPs). As any type of CMS survey proceeds, the coordinator must recognize the indications of how the survey is proceeding, and what must be done to minimize any errors or misinterpretations of fact. Having knowledge of the process—including what the surveyors will want to see—and being able to reasonably establish the outcome of the survey for the hospital and respond to survey findings are all critical elements of the survey coordinator's role.

CHAPTER 1

Know your surveyor

Know your surveyor

As survey coordinator, it is extremely important to understand the background and thinking of the surveyor or survey team when they arrive at your facility. Most surveyors come from state health agencies that contract with CMS to perform surveillance functions. Keep in mind that these individuals report to other state officials. That means you may have some recourse "locally," which should be used if there are points of contention over survey findings. Don't call your regional CMS office over a disagreement in regulatory interpretation until you have exhausted your efforts at the state level.

In some cases, you may find that the survey is being conducted by CMS itself. This is CMS' choice, and often may happen if:

- State resources are limited

- There is a specific complaint that interests CMS

- CMS audits state survey findings

Yes, CMS will survey a facility after state representatives have conducted a survey themselves. Although groans may arise from administration over this, it is vitally important to be on your guard if this specific situation occurs. It is within the purview of CMS to audit its state surveillance agencies (a "look-behind" survey). If this does happen, it may be a simple quality assessment of the state surveillance process. As sometimes happens, state surveyors may be accompanied by CMS representatives in a joint survey process. In any event, it is important to understand that surveyors may be influenced by the other surveys they conduct.

Survey staff may have a very wide range of surveillance experience. They are often called upon to be "generalists," covering all types of CMS-required surveillance from long-term care, home health care, renal dialysis centers, and, of course, acute care. Each variety of CMS-certified entity mentioned above has its own unique survey characteristics and requirements. In addition, the emphasis placed by CMS on those areas may transfer over to your hospital survey. It should not, but make sure you're knowledgeable about the CoPs and especially the Interpretive Guidelines that direct the surveyors. Although the surveyors may not have had recent (or any) acute-care experience, they have the Interpretive Guidelines to follow. Making yourself readily available to surveyors to answer questions or clarify their questions may prevent misinterpretation of hospital practices. Any hospital with a skilled nursing facility that is surveyed under the CoPs for long-term care will understand the dramatic difference between the two surveys. Long-term care is very prescriptive, and oriented toward certain specific outcome measures. For example, occurrence of decubitus ulcers and urine odor are two red flags for surveyors, and may lead to imposition of an immediate jeopardy as well as the possibility of losing Medicare reimbursement to the facility.

In the case of survey processes involving the *Life Safety Code® (LSC),* state surveyors are usually certified by CMS. In some states, the state fire marshal's representative conducts this portion of the survey. They may or may not have acute-care exposure with reference to these surveys. In any event, your facilities management staff should be prepared with the following:

- Any architectural drawings or plans for the hospital (or Statement of Condition in a Joint Commission-accredited hospital)

- The plans should clearly indicate smoke compartments and locations of exits

- If changes have been made to the facility structure, drawings should be available for those as well

Remember that the majority of deficiencies found on CMS surveys are found in the life-safety and environmental areas. Preparation for and involvement in the survey process will be critical for those department heads.

Know your survey

Know your survey

First, let's briefly recap the four types of CMS surveys:

Full survey

This is what the name implies—a full evaluation of the facility using the CoPs. These types of surveys are reserved for nonaccredited hospitals. The state agency or CMS schedules these within the window of the CMS fiscal year. However, your facility will not be made aware of the survey dates. Nonaccredited hospitals can expect to be surveyed every three years; the period for a hospital to be surveyed following nonaccreditation can be as short as 30–60 days after the date nonaccreditation becomes effective.

Sample validation survey

This is either a full survey of an accredited hospital or a partial survey of designated CoPs. It is commonly considered a "look-behind" survey. State agency surveyors do not need to see or hear a report on what problems or issues the accrediting surveyors found; they are in the facility to determine hospital compliance with the CoPs.

These surveys often come as a surprise to an accredited facility, since most are conducted within 60 days (and soon to be 30 days) immediately after the accrediting organization has conducted its survey. The purpose of these surveys is not necessarily to compare the accrediting agency's findings and CMS CoP compliance. It is primarily to determine that accrediting bodies effectively identify deficiencies in hospital operations and monitor corrective actions. The accredited hospitals selected for the look-behind validation surveys are approximately 1% of the accredited facilities annually. CMS has stepped up implementation of sample validations as a result of a critical Office of Inspector General report in July 1999, and has also reinstituted a "mid-cycle" validation of accredited hospitals 18 months after the accreditation survey.

With the move to unannounced surveys by the Joint Commission, these sample validation surveys may now be a little less troublesome, but the 30-day period following completion of the accreditator's survey is when this sample validation most likely will take place. The eighteenth month following an accrediting survey also bears watching.

Allegation survey

These surveys originate due to a number of factors, and can involve surveys of one or more (up to all) of the CoPs. The most common cause is a complaint against a facility filed with the federal government. This can be a letter or call to a federal elected or appointed representative by a constituent, or an anonymous complaint from any source. Quality Improvement Organizations (QIOs) which were formerly known as peer review organizations, may also be a source of referral to CMS for complaints. Finally, state agencies may refer complaints they receive to CMS, and in turn receive a directive from CMS to perform a survey. It is important to note that the complaint does not have to involve a Medicare or Medicaid recipient for a survey to be initiated. Any complaint, regardless of the complaint's source of insurance or lack thereof, may be investigated.

The complaint is reviewed, and the allegations regarding alleged misconduct are categorized and compared to the CoPs. CMS staff will then select the most applicable CoPs, and send a request to the state agency for a survey of those CoPs.

Emergency Medical Treatment and Active Labor Act (EMTALA, or antidumping) surveys are a type of allegation survey, and may involve not only review of compliance with the EMTALA CoP, but also the Emergency Services and Quality Assurance and Performance Improvement (QAPI) CoPs, to name two possibilities.

One final source of an allegation survey may be negative publicity. A report of an untoward event in the media, rumors of financial insolvency, or problems with another federal agency (such as Housing and Urban Development, the Internal Revenue Service, or the Drug Enforcement Administration) may ultimately find their way to CMS and a resultant survey request.

Distinct units

It is important to note that CoPs exist for acute care–certified rehabilitation or psychiatric units for which Prospective Payment System (PPS) waivers have been granted by CMS. In years past, state agencies were obliged to survey these units annually for compliance with the applicable CoPs. More recently, facilities complete an annual self-attestation of compliance, and no on-site survey is conducted. However, CMS may pick a sample of these units to be surveyed every year. As of 2004, facilities selected for a full validation survey will automatically have the distinct unit(s) CoPs reviewed for compliance by the survey team. This means those units, which previously were fairly untouched during a validation survey or full survey, will be extensively reviewed. The only exception to this policy is if the survey time frame falls within 90 days of the end of the federal cost-reporting period.

TIP: Always know what type of survey is being performed! Your survey response process should address each type of survey and the extent to which you need to marshal resources to respond.

CMS survey myths

Now, let's touch upon some CMS survey myths, and dispel any misunderstandings:

- MYTH: If surveyors don't have current acute-care backgrounds, their findings will be invalid or suspect.

REALITY: Nothing could be further from the truth. Remember that survey findings are based on the minimum standards in the CoPs. As one very experienced CEO once told me, "you don't have to be a CEO to interpret those standards." They may see something that you have always assumed to be right and proper. If you think about the findings, you may find that changes (i.e., corrections) are needed.

- MYTH: We can refute the deficiencies and stop any problems.

REALITY: You can discuss findings with the surveyors, and yes, you can disagree. But spending time refuting deficiencies may get you nowhere. If you spend time trying to make your case, you should think carefully about the what the effect will be if your arguments are not accepted. You may wind up having to quickly implement corrective action when you could have mollified the surveyors with an immediate positive response. Save arguments for after the survey, but give clarification and assistance to the surveyors immediately if you believe they are misinterpreting what you do.

- MYTH: We have no control over the surveyors, so they will find whatever they want and we'll just have to live with it.

REALITY: You can have control over what happens to your facility in a survey. The keys are as follows:

1. Survey preparation: Be prepared and be in compliance.

2. Understand the CoPs and make sure staff understand them.

3. Accompany the surveyors if at all possible, and watch what they see, hear, and do.

4. Intercede to prevent misunderstandings. Communicate frequently with the surveyor or survey team.

5. Even if the survey appears to be going badly, learn to develop positive, action-based responses. Although it may not affect the outcome, you can mitigate future problems.

Let's take a moment and cover the actions necessary in the last myth mentioned above:

1. Be prepared and in compliance.

Your facility should always be in compliance with the CoPs. That's the attitude and policy of CMS, and you need to adopt it to your institution. Not keeping up with the regulations, particularly if your hospital is non-accredited, is unforgivable!

Compliance is always difficult, particularly if you are Joint Commission–accredited and a CMS survey team shows up. Suddenly, your facility is faced with "new" standards and interpretations. Which ones do you follow? The answer, which you may not like, is BOTH. Products such as the *CMS-Joint Commission Crosswalk, 2008 Edition*, published by HCPro, can provide assistance in maintaining compliance in both areas.

2. Understand the CoPs and make sure staff understand them.

At the risk of being redundant, you must understand the CMS CoPs. These are available in an easy-to-reference format from HCPro, or can be found online. Included in this book is a handy reference to different federal Web sites for up-to-date information on the CoPs. Visit them often to monitor changes to the regulations and to see what may be approaching in regard to new requirements.

In the appendix, I've also included some enjoyable ways to get managers and staff members to understand CoPs that may affect them. The Quality Assurance and Performance Improvement CoP should be especially reviewed for pertinence to each department and service in the hospital.

3) **Accompany the surveyors if at all possible, and watch what they see, hear, and do.**

Never leave surveyors to their own devices or on their own in your facility unless they specifically request it. As they progress to each department or service, someone should anticipate their arrival and be there to greet them. That person should be a point person for that department. Remember surveys are unannounced and can occur when your department heads are on vacation. Designate backup staff beforehand in the event this happens. Unit nursing directors can be excellent persons to use when the nursing director is on vacation. Where situations like this are not possible, it may fall upon the survey coordinator to cover for that service or department. I don't recommend this as it ties up the coordinator in dealing with a specific area and may prevent him or her from seeing the broader picture of the survey from the perspective of the surveyors.

Surveyors will definitely want to have time alone to discuss their findings and arrange for completion of the survey process. Respect their need by providing a single location for them to meet, along with a phone for contact purposes. Always have a list of staff who they can contact in each department or service, and don't hesitate to contact those staff on your own if necessary. You might be able to prep the staff before the surveyors arrive, because as survey coordinator you should have an idea of where the survey is heading, and how the information from all the departments and services affected may be turning into deficiencies.

Watch what is happening in each area, every day the survey continues. Listen to the questions and answers between surveyors and staff. It may tell you something about what the surveyor is looking for, or where deficiencies may lie. In an allegation survey, this may give you an idea of what the complaint or problem is that was reported to CMS, and accordingly develop a response.

This also goes to what I mentioned at the introduction. You can control the survey by expediting what they need and clearing the process of any obstructions. Department head can't come in? Arrange a teleconference. Can't find a document? Have someone else search for it and get back to ensuring the survey continues on without interruption, or your presence.

4) **Intercede to prevent misunderstandings. Communicate frequently with the surveyor or survey team.**

It is important that the survey coordinator understand what is happening on each service or department as the survey progresses. Since the survey coordinator is usually one person, it becomes critical for the point person in each service or department to respond to the surveyors when they need answers or assistance, and that the information communicated is summarized to the survey coordinator. If something is stated incorrectly, make sure you contact the surveyors to correct the misunderstanding. In addition, you should ask for periodic updates from the survey staff, although they may wish to provide such only at the exit conference.

In any event, even if you only ask them how they are you doing and whether they need anything, that may be the most important action of the entire survey. You should check with them at least twice a day, unless they direct you otherwise. As mentioned above, if you keep the process moving, you should see the survey completed in the least amount of time necessary, or desired.

5) **Even if the survey appears to be going badly, learn to develop positive, action-based responses. Although it may not affect the outcome, it will mitigate future problems.**

Always start corrective action the minute you know a surveyor has detected a problem. They may not tell you if it is a deficiency or not, but if they mention it, you can bet it is at least of concern to them. Also, knowing the CoPs as I noted above will help you know if a deficiency is being identified.

Know the Conditions of Participation

Know the Conditions of Participation

This chapter offers tips on compliance with the hospital CoPs.

482.2 Provision of Hospital Services by Nonparticipating Hospitals

This is self-explanatory and is a means for hospitals that do not have Medicare provider agreements to receive Medicare and Medicaid reimbursement. Note that each bullet in the Interpretive Guidelines (IGs) must be met in order for those services to be billed. In the case of the last bullet, make sure you check with your state's licensing agency, should there be one, to determine if there are additional requirements in your state for a hospital to provide emergency services.

482.11 Compliance with federal, state and local laws

There are several components of this condition, which are important. First, note that the CEO or designees of the hospital may be asked to disclose whether any federal agencies have taken action against the facility. The surveyor may or may not seek out this information, but you should be prepared to discuss it, indicating at the same time any corrective action that was necessary. The example provided in the CoP (denying access to persons with disabilities) is simply one possible scenario. Failure to report medical equipment malfunctions to the Food and Drug Administration, or even violations of the Occupational Safety and Health Administration could be construed under this heading. In my experience, surveyors did not have such information prior to a survey. However, if there is an allegation (complaint) survey which was triggered by an unreported event mandated by federal law, be prepared to discuss what happened and how it is being prevented from recurring.

The other component of this CoP is the compliance issue with state and local laws. There was a fair amount of discussion over the years about the application of state and local laws to this requirement. Often, a facility might find itself cited on a CMS survey for violating state or local laws. Note that the IGs clearly address compliance with federal requirements, and direct the surveyors to report any violations such as those noted above to the appropriate federal agency. Usually, if a state agency is conducting the survey, CMS will want that referral routed through it, and may ask surveyors to conduct follow-up visits with the appropriate federal agency to determine the causes of the violation. A hospital should question a citation where only a violation of state or local law is cited, and there is no concomitant federal regulation to support such a citation.

482.11 (b)

This element requires a facility to be licensed in the state within which it is operating. This is self-explanatory.

482.11 (c)

This element requires those hospital staff members who require licensure or permits and/or other specialized training in the state to be duly accredited. It is important that your personnel office have evidence of appropriate licensure, permit, and/or training for any affected staff members as needed. You should insure that these credentials are up to date, and that a system is in place to identify those staff members who may not be currently licensed. Some states allow verification through official Web sites. Surveyors may then accept this as primary source verification for licensure, depending on state rules or policy.

Note particularly in the IGs that any practitioner engaged in telemedicine services must be licensed in the state in which the services are being provided. This includes offshore entities which may involve the use of foreign nationals. Like it or not, these individuals must possess appropriate licensing, and they should also have some form of credentialing as they may be performing medical services normally part of any hospital's medical staff structure. Remember to have a quality assurance/performance improvement (QAPI) program for these services as well.

482.12 Governing Body

The governing body is the primary entity responsible for all services provided. The recent emphasis in the corporate world concerning the governing body's knowledge and responsibility for the actions of its CEO—and in the case of hospitals, its medical staff—cause this Condition to be noteworthy for any hospital undergoing a survey. The new QAPI condition links the governing body to the assessment of the patient-care process. Exercising due diligence with respect to its financial and corporate responsibilities remains important as well.

Note that the IGs require the identity of a sole governing body responsible for operation of the hospital. For corporately managed or multiple-site facilities, there must be an identifiable body or individual responsible for operation of the facility. Facilities should be able to present surveyors with a clear, understandable organizational chart that shows how the governing body exercises its authority and fulfills its responsibilities for operation of the facility, including credentialing and assessment of the quality of care provided.

482.12 (a), (a) (1), and (a) (2) Medical Staff

The governing body is the sole entity that identifies and categorizes the practitioners who may render medical services in the facility. These categories must also be consistent with state laws governing the limits of practice for those individuals. This process is often identified in the governing-body bylaws, and is carried through into the medical staff bylaws. The governing body, as the ultimate authority for credentialing decisions, must ensure that there is evidence it assesses the medical staff's recommendations and does not simply act as a "rubber stamp" for the medical staff. Be careful with temporary privileging with respect to the appointment of medical staff members without some form of governing-body approval. Although the CEO may be vested to sign off on such appointments, it does not allow the governing body to abrogate its responsibility for ensuring that the proposed member meets all requirements of medical staff membership, and is in good standing with state authorities with respect to licensure.

(a) (3) and (4) Medical Staff Bylaws

Medical staff bylaws must be approved by the governing body, be consistent with state laws governing the credentialing process, and note that the CoP requires them to meet the CoPs. Ensure that the QAPI program and other elements such as the assessment of restraints by the medical staff are consistently met. Failure to do so may result in a citation with respect to lack of effective oversight.

Make sure any amendments or changes to the medical staff bylaws are properly annotated with the approval of the governing body and the date of approval. As always, the governing body should conspicuously follow its own bylaws with respect to approvals of any medical staff bylaws, rules, and regulations. The governing body is the final authority and responsible entity for appointments to the medical staff.

(a) (5)

As noted above, the medical staff's role in the QAPI program is identified here. Lack of an ongoing, effective program will lead to a citation here as well as under the CoP for QAPI.

(a)(6) & (7)

These last two elements go to ensuring that the governing body considers all the characteristics listed for membership to the medical staff. Again, a mere rubber-stamp approval will lead to problems down the road, particularly if the CMS survey team is in your hospital because of the misadventures of one of the medical staff members.

482.12 (b) Chief Executive Officer

This element is self-explanatory.

482.12 (c)

This element is self-explanatory, but it should be noted that a clinical psychologist may care for a Medicare patient, consistent with state law, but within the limits of the practice of clinical psychology. A patient with concomitant medical problems will also need the intervention of a licensed independent practitioner (LIP) where necessary.

482.12 (c) (1) through (c) (4)

These elements discuss the care of patients under CMS regulation, including the responsibilities of practitioners. As mentioned above, note that granting admission privileges for LIPs does not abrogate the responsibility of a physician to be present to address a patient's problems that fall within the physician's purview.

482.12 (d) Standard: Institutional Plan and Budget

(1 through 7)

This standard includes two important requirements:

- The existence of an operating budget, prepared and approved by the governing body. A committee of the governing body may do the preparation and must include representation from administration and the medical staff of the hospital.

- This also calls for the establishment of a capital expenditure plan (or budget) which is projected for a three-year period. One of those three years must be the current year. Any capital expenditure, which may be part of a formal certificate of need application to a state, must be subject to their approval.

Both budgets must be approved and, in the case of the capital budget, reviewed annually. Some hospitals that are non-accredited may make this decision based on the cost of an accreditation survey. The challenges of operating on a daily basis may cause the facility to lose sight of its capital needs. This should not be the case, as surveyors cannot grant a pass-through for noncompliance with this standard.

482.12 (e) Contracted Services

This is an important standard that may be misunderstood. It requires the oversight of contracted services by the hospital, including the assessment of these services by the hospital's QAPI program. The extent to which all services should be evaluated may be in question (e.g., groundskeeping services under contract). However, a common flaw is to have physician contract services not evaluated, particularly where these services may be rendered by a sole practitioner (e.g., pathology services) or by a physician group (e.g., radiology or emergency services). Hospitals mistakenly have no peer review for the sole-practitioner scenario, or have only the hospital-based QAPI program for departments like radiology. In the case of the sole practitioner, some form of peer review by another cooperating practitioner in the area can actually help both facilities accomplish this end. For the radiology scenario, a peer-review program should be in place to ensure accuracy (i.e., overreading) of radiology reports.

In any event, it is important to have a written inventory of contracted services, and to be able to determine the extent to which they provide or affect your patient care. If they do, make sure their services are included in your QAPI program.

482.12 (f) Emergency Services

In these days of Emergency Medical Treatment and Active Labor Act (EMTALA) violations, it is important to ensure the hospital remains compliant with the applicable provision of the Emergency Services CoP.

This Condition simply refers back to the CoP for Emergency Services in that respect. Note, however, that it goes on to explain the need for reacting to emergency care situations in all off-site and on-site locations. In other words, simply calling "911" will not suffice when a patient has a cardiac arrest in your internal medicine off-site clinic. Although it may be part of the staff's response to such an event, there should be policies and procedures consistent with the services provided in that clinic to address how the patient may be treated pending the arrival of EMS or other staff to treat the patient's emergency condition. EMTALA addresses this issue as one of capacity; in other words, it would not be expected that the patient would receive full life-sustaining treatment if a cardiac arrest occurred in an off-site physical therapy clinic where no physicians are present.

Nonetheless, staff should be trained and familiar with the policies and procedures to address such an emergency. It would be reasonable to expect that as surveyors visit off-site clinics, this will be an area of interest. Hospital "ownership" of services is determined by whether there are any services billed by the hospital to Medicare. The sites of those services must comply with this requirement.

482.13 Patients' Rights

This CoP is a recent and, in some cases, controversial addition to the CoPs. During a survey, it would be expected to be coordinated by one surveyor, most likely an RN from the survey team. Note that the CoP requires the ongoing provision of information to a patient in order for them to make informed decisions concerning their care and posthospital needs. Note especially the elements in bold under the IG for 482.13(a)(1). Note also that it is expected that the patient will understand any form of communication. Every attempt should be made to ensure the patient both receives and understands his or her rights as a Medicare patient. Although this regulation does not mandate the documentation of proof that these rights have been provided, good practice would dictate a simple check-off at the time of admission that such rights were provided (or could not be provided immediately due to emergency circumstances). At some point surveyors will be asking patients to show they learned of their rights in the hospital. Although this process may be flawed (e.g., patients can't recall, or think they may not have received their rights when they were admitted), the surveyors may use a more global analysis to determine of there is a trend towards patients not receiving their rights, such as a series of patients interviewed who state they have no idea what their rights are.

482.13 (a) (2) Grievances

CMS expects hospitals to have an effective way of dealing with complaints from patients or others. This section defines the grievance process to be a complaint about patient care, and one that cannot be resolved on the spot. A policy and procedure should be in place, and understood by the staff, describing how patient complaints must be handled. Billing complaints are not considered grievances, so the focus is on patient care. Note especially that the governing body must approve the grievance process. Make sure that the approval has not been delegated off to the patient advocate or administration. If your state has a provision for its own set of patient's rights and/or a grievance procedure, ensure that the patient is aware of this also. State laws may allow the patient to file a grievance with the state. This information and the procedure for doing so must be offered to the patient if he or she does not wish to deal with the hospital or if he or she is unhappy with the facility's investigation.

As interviews are conducted, it will be important that patients are at least able to access some written material provided by the hospital about their rights and the grievance process. As long as something is available at the patient's bedside, it will cover much of what the surveyors may expect to see.

482.13 (b) Exercise of Rights

This standard spells out the expectations for hospitals with reference to patients' ability to participate in their plans of care. Note the reference to the patients' participation in their pain management plans, which has received heavy focus from many state agencies as well as the Joint Commission and now CMS. You should ensure that this is a key component of your overall patient management plan, and your pharmacy and therapeutics (P&T) committee as well as your nursing leadership should carefully develop this plan in accord with current standards of care. As always, this should be a proactive process, as noted in the standard, and not a process created after the patient is in pain and cannot give meaningful input.

Also contained in this standard is the right of the patient to be informed of choices with reference to post-discharge care. In some cases, large organizations which have a wide range of postdischarge services available (e.g., nursing home, home health, hospice) may wish to refer the patient into that network only. Facilities should be careful in making such decisions so as not to violate the patient's freedom of choice. Failure to do so could possibly violate CMS or state requirements.

The standard also addresses the patient's right to choose or refuse treatment, consistent with law. Your policies should address potential conflicts and include intervention by hospital legal counsel when necessary.

Advance directives are also addressed, and in some states there are statutes or regulations addressing advance directives. Very simply, the patient has the right, consistent with law, to make decisions regarding life-sustaining treatment. Surveyors will look for facility notification to inpatients (some states may require notice to all patients) regarding their right to make such directives, usually at the time treatment is initiated. Note that the IGs for this standard require the surveyor to ask what education has been provided to both staff and patients over the planning for and/or implementation of an advance directive.

482.13 (c) Standard: Privacy and Safety

We will not cover the elements of the Health Insurance Portability and Accountability Act in this section, but you should have stringent policies already in place. The federal Office of Civil Rights is currently enforcing these standards. However, note that this standard asks some key questions of the surveyor in the IGs. The storage of patient charts outside the room (either in door containers or on med carts) can possibly be seen to violate this standard. Also, the placement of names on med sheets or precaution sheets on the door may also violate this standard. If it has not already been done, facility policies and procedures should be in place to address this. The patient-care staff and especially the medical staff must be keenly aware of the need for patient privacy in the institution.

The requirements held forth in section c (2) are especially important in these times, and deserve special consideration. Your facility should have an overall patient-safety program in place. It should be linked to the QAPI program, and be part of both the medical staff and hospital-based programs.

Security is important and must be balanced with the privacy of the patient. Incident and accident reports will be reviewed and should reflect findings, conclusions, and actions taken to prevent further problems. Continuous evidence of patient falls should be addressed vigorously, and the incidence reduced or preferably eliminated. Failure to do so will result in an extended survey and more questions by the surveyors, and ultimately citations.

The standard also goes on to address patient abuse. These requirements may sound familiar to hospitals who have nursing homes subject to CMS survey. Since your CMS survey team may also have experience completing nursing-home surveys, you should pay attention to this standard. Refer to the components necessary for abuse prevention, and be able to provide surveyors with some policies and procedures from patient-care staff members which show how abuse is prevented. Be careful that staff members avoid inadvertent abuse by verbal or other-than-physical means. Ensure that your nursing staff has an effective program in place for the identification, treatment, and ultimate prevention of bedsores (decubitus ulcers). Your survey team may focus on patients who come from the nursing-home environment where such problems are not to occur. If patients develop decubitus ulcers while in your facility, surveyors will undoubtedly focus on this.

482.13 (d) Standard: Confidentiality of Patient Records

As mentioned previously, confidentiality of records is important in the surveillance process. Your medical-records staff should be able to demonstrate how records are released to those legally allowed. The issue of confidentiality previously discussed when referring to active inpatient records is important as well. All your off-site locations should also be following the same policies and procedures for outpatient services confidentiality. It would be wise during the facility's mock-survey preparation to visit each off-site location to ensure they are compliant.

482.13 (e) Standard: Restraint for Acute Medical and Surgical Care, and (f) Standard: Seclusion and Restraint for Behavior Management

Here we see another similarity to long-term care and the nursing home–surveillance process. This has caused a fair degree of controversy, particularly with the frequency at which an LIP assesses a patient in restraints.

We are not going into detail concerning these standards for several reasons. First, they consume almost 50 pages of the IGs, which is remarkable in that the entire document is approximately 400 pages. Second, the detail given in the IGs should, for the most part, be self-explanatory. That being said, the following guidelines should be considered:

- Physical or chemical restraints or seclusion should be used sparingly or not at all. It is readily apparent that CMS is encouraging the use of restraints as a last-ditch modality of treatment.

- Any application of restraints or imposition of seclusion should follow strict internal policies. A prior-to-application review system to approve restraints or seclusion in noncritical situations would be recommended.

- As noted here, any patient who dies while in restraints/seclusion must be reported to CMS. This overrides any similar state law, and may thus require dual reporting to both CMS and the state. Do not assume that reporting to the state will suffice, and that the state will inform CMS. It is the facility's responsibility to notify CMS in the time frames indicated.

- Surveyors will be focusing on any patients receiving physical or chemical restraints, or who are in seclusion while a survey is being conducted. If your facility is a psychiatric hospital, or if your facility has a Prospective Payment System (PPS)–exempt psychiatric unit, ensure that any restrained/secluded patient has evidence of full justification and, as mentioned above, a form of approval through the facility's medical and nursing staff for the restraints.

- In the event of a death of a patient in restraints, immediately launch a full root-cause analysis, and determine why it happened. It may bring CMS to your door, particularly if there is negative publicity. Corrective action will in all probability be necessary, and should be implemented hospitalwide as soon as possible.

482.21 Condition of Participation: Quality Assessment and Performance Improvement

This is a new Condition that replaced the outdated Quality Assurance Condition about a year ago. The focus of this CoP is now oriented toward performance improvement for the entire facility. The emphasis is on the utilization of data in evaluation of quality, and taking a proactive approach to quality improvement. There are links in philosophy to the Joint Commission's recent emphasis on failure mode and effects analysis (FMEA). Both approaches call for the application of changes to systems before a problem occurs. The emphasis is away from individual case review to the aggregate analysis of data. For example, surgical complications can be reviewed individually for potential problems, but should also be trended to determine if the rate of complication for a given procedure is unacceptable.

This is CMS' reference to "projects" as a means of improvement. It should not infer that the projects should determine that there is an acceptable rate of complications. FMEA, which finds its basis in the aerospace program, is the analysis of a given repetitive system to determine how many times a system can function effectively before a breakdown will occur. Simply put, in a medical care system, how is the care system for prevention of a decubitus ulcer put in place by the nursing staff? What are the key stress points where that system can break down? This can be applied retrospectively in case review, but is most effective and meant for review BEFORE any problem occurs. This will require those hospitals that may not have been caught up in performance improvement over the years to reassess their quality-review programs. Case review will no longer be the sole determinant of compliance. It will be up to your QAPI staff to implement this program and keep it effective. Likewise, the need for reduction of medical error requires the review of data and the analysis of the systems of care before untoward events occur.

482.21 (a) Standard: Program Scope

This standard lays the basis for the CoP, and the expectation that a hospital, through conduct of studies, will be able to show *measurable* improvement in both healthcare outcomes, and in reduction of medical error. Since this CoP is still relatively new, there have not been formal IGs issued. However, surveyors have been issued interim guidelines and will expect facilities to be fully compliant. Here are the highlights of this CoP and what you should be doing to comply:

- The governing body and the executive staff are responsible for ensuring that the program is effectively implemented and maintained. Note that the executive staff members are expected to provide whatever resources are necessary to ensure the program analyzes and prevents the potential causes of medical error. This will include the proper staffing of your QAPI program. An experienced staff member with QAPI background will be able to work with your medical director and your hospital-based departments to ensure the identification of meaningful indicators and relevant data. Because these staff members seemingly do not generate revenue, they tend to be the first to be cut back or have additional responsibilities assigned such as discharge planning or infection control. This is not prohibited, however, if any citations are identified, the failure may be attributed to a lack of sufficient support for the QAPI program by the executive staff and/or the governing body.

- Many current quality-assurance/improvement programs do have indicators which are assessed to determine the frequency of either a negative or positive occurrence in the provision of patient care. This CoP calls for an in-depth assessment of these indicators. Many programs have a tendency to simply report the frequency of occurrence on a monthly or quarterly basis, and then at the end of the report state "continue to monitor." The idea of data assessment is to move toward improvement or lessening of these occurrences by analyzing frequency, time of occurrence, severity of event and so on. If indicators are not occurring with any particular frequency or severity, this CoP indicates you should look at something else in order to improve care.

- The data collection and analysis **do not** remove the responsibility for effective peer review, or root cause analysis (RCA) once an incident occurs. It is critical to ensure that these mechanisms remain in place. Even the best proactive QAPI program will not prevent the occurrence of a medical error. An effective RCA process will address the event and implement solutions which then may be assessed for identification of indicators for inclusion into the QAPI program.

482.21 (a) and (b) Program Scope and Program Data

The outline for meeting this CoP is addressed here. Note that the governing body must formulate and approve the QAPI program, as well as the frequency and detail of data collection. The program must include indicators, including adverse patient events. It is recommended that any *potential* adverse event be clearly identified as an indicator. If your program fails to identify an event, you may find CMS in your facility investigating the occurrence and find that it was not reviewed by your QAPI program.

482.21 (c) Program Standards

This standard requires the tracking of medical errors, determining their incidence, and developing strategies for their elimination. It is important to note here that medical errors should not be construed as solely within the domain of the medical staff, nor only significant patient-care incidents. A surveyor could easily determine that the occurrence of decubitus ulcers is too frequent in your facility, and may ask what your QAPI program has done to address this. Although this may not be the traditional definition of medical error, their occurrence may be considered something that should not be happening. In that sense, it can be classified as an adverse patient event. Failure of a patient to achieve his or her goals in a rehabilitation program could be considered an adverse patient outcome. The patient didn't achieve his or her goals. Why? What is the frequency of patients not achieving their rehab goals? Are there enough staff members to ensure that goals are met? These are the kinds of naturally progressing questions that a surveyor may ask. All of this may be found during the patient interview process by survey staff. Your QAPI program should have the answers.

Note that the QAPI program must have sufficient depth to deal with the scope and complexity of services offered in the hospital. A small rural hospital will have a less complex program than a large urban facility. However, a rehab unit in a rural hospital will deserve the same amount of program (at least as a baseline) as attributed to a large urban facility.

482.21 (d) Performance Improvement Projects

The standard defines the projects as annual, but there is no prohibition to their being less than annual, or ongoing. The point here is to ensure the identification of measures on a timely basis to improve care and effectively implement them. Note that hospitals may develop an information technology system to assist in this process. The standard allows a "pass" for a hospital to develop this system without immediately demonstrating improvement in the indicators being measured. However, this is a one-time event, and surveyors will expect that the system will be up and running upon their return. Hospitals should be able to provide surveyors with a timetable for implementation of the system including production of data and time frames for implementing indicator improvement where possible.

Also, hospitals may participate in a program developed by the QIO in the hospital's designated geographic area. The hospital can weigh its involvement in such a project or choose to develop its own. The project must be comparable to the QIO's scope of evaluation.

(e) Executive Responsibilities

As mentioned previously, hospital executive staff bears a large part of the responsibility for implementation of the QAPI program. The resources necessary to fuel this program are a direct responsibility of the executive staff. The improvement projects are also required to be conducted annually.

482.22 Condition of Participation: Medical Staff

The medical staff of a hospital is expected to be one body, not several. For multiple-site locations which are part of a system with one Medicare provider number, a single medical staff is expected. Although their assignments may be to different campuses or levels of care, it is still expected that their primary membership exists on the one medical staff.

482.22 (a) Standard: Composition of the Medical Staff

(1) and (2)

These elements require the examination of credentials for those staff members seeking reappointment to the medical staff, as well as new appointments. Notice that the IGs mention an "outcome-oriented" appraisal system for members being recredentialed. This feeds from the results of peer review. As earlier indicated, do not forget the value of peer review for assessing renewal of staff privileges.

For new candidates, the system for appointment should follow the medical staff bylaws. To repeat, the governing body is the final determinant as to privileges. The system must ensure the presence of current licensure and/or certification, and also determine if there is sufficient compliance with any additional state requirements for licensure at initial application and for renewal. This would include any mandatory continuing education or training.

482.22 (b) Standard: Medical Staff Organization and Accountability and (c) Medical Staff Bylaws

These standards are self-explanatory. The leadership of the medical staff may be assigned to the medical executive committee (MEC) or to the medical director or president of the medical staff in concert with the MEC. A formal structure should exist for organization of the medical staff, regardless of the size of the institution. The medical staff should be aware of the leadership, and the governing body should ensure that it follows its own bylaws with respect to the medical staff. As an example, the medical director or chief of staff may be recognized as the individual responsible for the medical staff, but governing-body minutes may find the president (elected) of the medical staff presenting the staff's report to the governing body. Bylaws should be consistent with reality and vice versa.

All practitioners should have privileges assigned that outline the extent to which they may practice within the facility. Expect the surveyor to determine if surgeons are performing procedures consistent with their approved privileges, and that no surgical procedure may be performed without the privilege for that procedure being granted. The bylaws should be strictly followed, including a process for granting privileges for new procedures not previously performed at the hospital (such as bariatric surgery).

482.22 (c) (5) History and Physical Examinations

This element defines at length the requirements for a current history and physical (H&P) examination to be placed into the patient's chart. From time to time, CMS requirements may conflict with Joint Commission, American Osteopathic Association, or state requirements. When in doubt, make sure you are compliant with CMS standards. If there is a conflict, try to determine from your state agency the areas where compliance is necessary over and above the CMS requirements, and if a conflict exists, how they may allow your facility to meet both requirements. CMS will insist that their requirements supercede state requirements where conflicts exist, so keep that in mind. This is also true for Joint Commission requirements. If you have a CMS survey, and are cited for a compliance issue, do not use the reasoning that Joint Commission has a requirement that is different. You will be expected to comply with the CMS requirement first. CMS and the Joint Commission work closely to make the CoPs and Joint Commission standards as consistent as possible, and prevent these things from happening.

482.22 (d) Standard: Autopsies

This standard is a holdover from the previous 1980s-era CoPs. Nonetheless, it remains to be met by facilities. You should ensure that somewhere there is a defined policy on the securing and performance of autopsies, including the notification of the attending practitioner when one is performed. This might also include medical examiner cases where the death may be ruled "suspicious." The process for securing permission of the deceased patient's next of kin should be outlined in these procedures as well.

482.23 Condition of Participation: Nursing Services

The IGs for this Condition are now more distinct, and include the necessity of having the nursing services QAPI program integrated into the hospital's program. This does not mean the simple forwarding of reports into the hospitalwide program. It means the active participation of nursing staff with all levels of care in the hospital. It is suggested that the "Joint Conference Committee" used with the governing body and medical staff be extended to nursing services as well. An integrated committee with representatives of the medical staff, executive staff, and nursing staff could be a valuable means to address QAPI issues.

482.23 (a)

The organization of nursing should be reflected in an understandable organizational chart, utilizing as a reference (but not exactly) the position descriptions shown in the IGs. Any use of outside contract staff in nursing services must be represented in the chart and must be a component of nursing services supervision. As the IGs indicate, all nursing services must be under the purview of the hospital. A nurse working in a primary-care off-site clinic, for which the hospital bills Medicare, must be supervised by the nursing service of the hospital, not the physician(s) in the clinic.

482.23 (b) Standard: Staffing and Delivery of Care

There are important distinctions in staffing that should be addressed prior to the survey. Note that the IG for this standard requires "a registered nurse (RN) physically present on the premises and on duty at all times." The standard itself calls for the "immediate availability" of an RN for the care of a patient. The IG defines immediate availability and the restrictions associated with "floating" RN staff to the extent that an RN would be assigned to several floors. While this could be explained to surveyors if only one or two patients are on one floor, the risk associated with floating an RN to different floors may result in an adverse event, or inadequate patient care which may be picked up by the surveyors.

The standard also defines the utility of a licensed practical nurse (LPN) as long as the LPN is under the supervision of an RN. For rural hospitals, there are waiver provisions for the 24-hour nursing requirement found in this standard. Rural hospitals should seek this information utilizing reference to the CFR provisions mentioned.

There is no formula for staffing other than that shown in the standard. Surveyors may rely more heavily on patient interviews, any indications that care is not being provided on a timely basis, or care not within the standards of good nursing.

482.23 (b) (2)

This requires all nurses and (as mentioned earlier) any other nursing staff to be licensed. Your policies and procedures should demonstrate this in the manner previously outlined.

The standard goes on to identify the components of a nursing care plan and the need for registered nurses to supervise nursing care, including agency staff members. These may be utilized in nonaccredited hospitals as nursing indicators for the QAPI program, but must also relate to the provision of patient care and how care is *improved*. Keep that in mind as your nursing staff develops the QAPI program.

With reference to agency staff, note the requirements of the IGs relative to supervision of agency (i.e., non-hospital-employed) nurses, and the need for their supervision by a hospital-employed RN. The use of an agency nurse on nights to supervise staff members could be problematic if that person is unable to identify how he or she is supervised. There is no indication in the IGs that on-site supervision is necessarily required. Evaluation of an individual agency staff member's work performance must be completed annually, and must be available for the surveyor. Finally, ensure that the services provided by these staff members are part of the hospital's QAPI program.

482.23 (c) Standard: Preparation and Administration of Drugs

This standard is important in that there need to be defined methods for the administration of medication by the nursing staff. Since medication errors are one of the top adverse events occurring in healthcare, it is important for the facility and its medical staff to develop the medication administration policy, and for nursing to have an effective medication administration review component in the QAPI program. This can be handled through the facility's P&T process as a joint effort. Ensure that any staff members who are not RNs are administering medications, including the initiation of IV lines, in accordance with any state protocols, licensure, or registration. For example, some states may disallow radiological technicians from administering IV solutions. Make sure your nursing leadership has knowledge of the proper protocols involving nonnursing staff members.

482.23 (c) (2) (i-iii)

These elements deal with the issuance of verbal orders. Note the detail listed for the content of a verbal order. It is important that the practitioner understand his or her obligation for countersignature, and the need to use such orders sparingly. As a start, if the practitioner is in the facility, they should be asked to come back to the nurses' station to complete the order, rather than issuing it verbally. Be aware of Joint Commission or American Osteopathic Association requirements, as well as any state regulations governing these types of orders.

482.23 (c) (3)

The administration of transfusions and IV meds should be carefully controlled in accordance with licensure restrictions (if any) in your state, as well as good nursing practice. There should be evidence of distinct training for these services. For the sake of identification, each individual in each patient-care unit should be identified in writing on the unit as to their authorization to perform these procedures. The surveyor will probably want to see this material.

482.24 Condition of Participation: Medical Record Services

This CoP sets forth the standards for medical-record services. "Medical records" is broadly defined in the standards. Your medical-record department should be well prepared with records that are as complete as possible. Surveyors are required to review both active and closed records. The record review sample will vary according to hospital census, and will also include a portion of outpatient records.

The balance of the Conditions are self-explanatory in that they set forth common-sense organization and operation of the medical-records department, and also touch on elements of confidentiality and records release mentioned before. Your medical-record department should be secure, functioning efficiently, and, above all, be able to track medical-record delinquency on the part of the medical staff. Corrective action to deal with your facility's primary offenders should be taken before the problem gets out of control, and is noticed by survey staff. It may well lead them to ask if the facility's recredentialing process is effective when physicians continue to be reappointed despite significant medical-record delinquency.

The nature of medical-record authentication by the practitioner is also addressed at length. This includes electronic signatures. The timeframes for conducting H&Ps are again addressed in detail. Consents for treatment are covered and defined. These and the remaining requirements are clearly addressed and are self-explanatory.

482.25 Condition of Participation: Pharmaceutical Services

This CoP covers the organization and operation of the pharmacy services. These services must be under the direction of a registered pharmacist. Much of the initial part of this CoP discusses the need for prevention of medication errors. Particular attention should be given to the fact that review of medication errors is a responsibility of the hospital's pharmaceutical service. This function may be conducted under nursing services, but ultimately remains a responsibility of the pharmaceutical service. You should ensure that there is an organized review process to coordinate any medication-error review activities, including any FMEA studies. The long list of examples for study shows the level of federal interest in reducing one of the most common and potentially deadly forms of medical error. The medical staff must be be allied with this effort, either through the P&T review process, or some other means to ensure that any medical staff actions will be analyzed as well.

With reference to medication storage, management, and administration, your medication storage procedures must ensure the safety of the medications from diversion, a safe means of storage to protect medications from damage, and you must issue medications under the direction of a licensed pharmacist. The pharmacy must be managed by a licensed pharmacist, whether consultative or full time. In those situations where a consultant pharmacist is used, ensure that the pharmacist is actively involved in P&T functions with the medical staff, and that this consultative oversight is not merely a signoff of activities in the pharmacy department. Establish clear expectations, including the ongoing operation of the pharmacy QAPI program and evidence of ongoing dialogue with the medical staff. As noted in the IGs, actual supervision of the pharmacy will be reviewed. Do not limit the supervising pharmacist to an hour or two a month. Mere countersignatures on QAPI reports or pharmacy policies and procedures will not be sufficient as evidence of supervision. Only active involvement on a reasonably frequent basis, based on the scope and complexity of the services offered by the hospital, will suffice.

In addition, surveyors will examine whether or not there are sufficient numbers of pharmacy staff to provide pharmaceutical services at the hospital. Remember that the primary emphasis here is on safety and control of medication delivery. Lack of sufficient resources or evidence of high numbers of medication errors may lead not only back to nursing services, but also pharmacy oversight. Insufficient staffing may be cited if the pharmacist does not have the manpower to accomplish his or her responsibilities.

Note again the reference to "high-risk" medications and the resources available to identify these medications. The pharmacy should keep this list current, and high-risk meds should be an indicator in the QAPI program for review. It is strongly suggested that FMEA-type studies referenced earlier be instituted for these medications to determine possible error points in the distribution process. This can be shown to surveyors and will accomplish meeting the medication safety goal, as well as the assessment requirements of the QAPI condition.

482.25 (b) (2)

Pay attention to the issue of "locked" storage of medications, because it pertains to the medication carts on the floors that nursing staff use to distribute medications. It is very important to read the IG with reference to these carts, and the guidance for determining how nursing staff should handle distribution while keeping the carts secure. Hospitals have been cited because carts were left in hallways unlocked and unobserved while nursing staff members were distributing meds in patient rooms.

The standard goes on to cover the need for systems to ensure the removal of outdated mislabeled or otherwise unusable drugs. This should be readily apparent to surveyors on the floors. During a mock survey, your staff should conduct a medication review of drug cabinets, refrigerators, and so on. Are the refrigerators at the proper temperature?

Access to the pharmacy during off-hours should be restricted. What are the policies and procedures for acquisition of medications by nursing staff members during off-hours? If access is frequent, surveyors may question the adequacy of medication supply and storage facilities. The standard also defines the need for a medical staff–approved formulary system, which must be carefully monitored to assure cost-effectiveness, current applicability to services offered by the hospital, and especially to be supportive for the prevention of medication interaction.

The last section covers the need for analysis of adverse drug reactions, and the ongoing QAPI analysis of any medication errors.

Do not make the mistake of solely attributing medication errors to staff members. The standard clearly states the expectation that the medication delivery system will be reviewed when a med error occurs, and not merely a sanction against the staff member presumably responsible for the error.

482.26 Condition of Participation: Radiological Services

As this Condition indicates, the hospital must have the means to provide radiological services to its patients. Typically, the hospital provides the physical space, most of the equipment, and support and technical staff for these services. Often the professional component is under contract with a radiologist or group. More recently, physicians have offered to purchase newer types of technology in partnership with hospitals. As this intermix has matured, it is important for hospitals not to lose sight of the need for a hospital-based QAPI program in radiology. The technical quality-assurance aspects of radiation safety, calibration of equipment, and staff techniques are all-important aspects to be evaluated. However, short shrift is often given to the need for an effective professional component review in the QAPI program. Merely comparing ("overreading") radiology reports or films should not be considered the sole QAPI indicator. For example, a review program integrated with technical support staff will be important to prevent misadministration of contrast material, or excessive or insufficient administration of therapeutic radiation.

Ensure that all staff in your radiology service are properly credentialed and trained to administer radiological services consistent with their licensure and/or registration. Personnel files should clearly indicate up-to-date certification where necessary. In some states, there may be limitations on the ability of technicians to start IV contrast. Make sure your service is operating in accordance with state and federal standards.

As was mentioned previously, radiologists who provide radiology services must be licensed in the state in which the services are provided. You must have a credentials file for all providers of service, whether on site or not. Do not assume that a contracted group is not part of your medical staff if they provide radiology services. If they look like doctors and provide services like doctors, then they should be on your medical staff.

Keep in mind the requirement for signatures when reports are completed. Electronic signatures are subject to the provisions found in the Medical Records CoP, so refer to them to ensure you are in compliance.

482.27 Condition of Participation: Laboratory Services

We will not dwell at length on this CoP, as the IGs are quite comprehensive. Clinical Laboratory Improvement Amendments requirements are also addressed in the regulation and are pertinent to these standards. In some states, this Condition may be surveyed by a state laboratorian, or by an individual from a state agency responsible for laboratory certifications.

Be alert to the need for providing lab services 24 hours a day, seven days a week. Cost cutting may raise the desire to contract out services on weekends, or in their entirety. Remember to keep these requirements in mind when considering such actions. Note especially the emphasis in (c) on potentially infectious blood and blood products. The primary emphasis here is the existence of a "look-back" program to assess if an incident has occurred where a patient is transfused with "tainted" blood or blood products. A policy and procedure for the quarantining of potentially infected blood or blood products must be in existence for the surveyor to review.

482.28 Condition of Participation: Food and Dietetic Services

This Condition is seemingly straightforward. For the acute hospital, however, there are some elements which bear attention.

As mentioned before, some of the concepts of long-term care have entered into the acute CoPs. Most importantly, since surveyors are interviewing patients on your units, and will be reviewing their records, any indication that nutrition is inadequate will lead to citations. This would most likely occur when patients with special needs are assessed. Skin breakdowns or infections may be reviewed, and nutrition services will play a part in the care these patients receive. We mention this because we want to emphasize the patient-care aspect of nutrition management. There is enough in this Condition relative to safe food handling, storage, and general management of the dietary service.

For those facilities that have a food-service director who is not a dietitian, the qualifications are spelled out. Note that a dietitian is required, and is responsible for the nutritional needs of patients under the hospital's care. It is important that these two individuals coordinate nutritional care, but the responsibility for assessing and ensuring these needs are met belongs to the dietitian.

482.30 Condition of Participation: Utilization Review

For the most part, this CoP will not be surveyed as long as the hospital has an agreement with a designated QIO, which acts as the review agent for various localities throughout the country. You can check with your regional CMS office or your local Medicare Fiscal Intermediary if you are unsure. The balance of the requirements found in this Condition are self-explanatory. Make sure you have copies available of any utilization review agreements with a designated QIO or review agent.

482.41 Condition of Participation: Physical Environment

We have mentioned previously the need to have certain documents ready for a survey. For this CoP, you should have a full set of building plans for all sites, both inpatient and outpatient. These plans should indicate types of materials used in construction, dates of construction and any additions, and floor plans with designated smoke compartments.

In addition, your Facility Operations staff should have evidence of an effective QAPI program that addresses ongoing evaluation of the suitability of the environment and the level of safety needed to protect patients. Note the section in the IGs relative to emergency preparedness. Most states have direction from federal authorities as to the roles that hospitals may play in both local and national emergencies. Your disaster preparedness plan should take into account both internal and external emergencies, as well as the need for any external assistance or coordination. Although there are no specific requirements within the standards for the makeup of a major disaster plan, you should closely coordinate with your local emergency management authorities to ensure you will not only be able to assist them, but that in a disaster your facility will in turn receive the attention it will need to function effectively.

Where necessary, you should also contact the Federal Emergency Management Agency to determine any other needs that may not be addressed. Some questions to ask are as follows:

- Does the facility have a sufficient source of potable water in the event of a termination of water supplies?

- Does the facility have access to sufficient fuel supplies to power its emergency generator(s)?

482.41 (b) Standard: Life Safety from Fire

This standard may be surveyed by any of a number of different entities, depending on how your state certifies health-facility compliance for fire safety. Some state agencies employ their own life safety specialists, while some will delegate this to the local fire marshal. The entity in charge of surveying life safety is based on the "authority having jurisdiction" concept. The facility should check state or local laws to determine who has jurisdiction and who will conduct this portion of the survey. CMS now mandates compliance with the year 2000 edition of the *Life Safety Code® (LSC)*issued by the National Fire Protection Association (NFPA). Remember that outpatient locations for which the hospital bills its services must also meet these codes. Now that surveyors are mandated to evaluate outpatient facilities more thoroughly, careful preparation with your facilities management staff should be maintained. As noted further on in the standard, if the state has equivalent laws which meet fire safety standards, then CMS may accept these as equivalent to their life safety requirements. Again, check with your state to determine this.

This standard contains a provision for waivers from *LSC* requirements, if it can be shown that the strict imposition of the standards would result in an "unreasonable hardship" for a facility. The application process for a waiver will be either through your state agency, or CMS. If the aforementioned state standards are in effect instead of CMS' requirements, you may not be able to obtain a waiver.

When filing for a waiver, it is best to discuss it with an architect or fire-safety consultant to determine if the chances of an *LSC* waiver being granted are good. Do not assume that being unable to comply automatically will lend itself to approval. You may have to "jump through hoops" to get a waiver approved, and there is no guarantee that it will be accepted.

Finally, note the requirement to meet the roller-latch standard for doors, and the 90-minute requirement for emergency lighting.

The balance of the standard is self-explanatory with the help of the IGs.

482.41 (b) Standard: Facilities

The IGs cover the survey requirements well. Ensure that there are no storage issues with equipment or supplies that compromise fire safety. This includes the placement of extraneous equipment like chairs, beds, gurneys, IV machines, etc., in hallways, and especially in stairwells or other areas of ingress or egress. Also supplies should be safely stored—at least 18 inches from the ceiling in sprinklered areas, and off the floor to ensure proper cleaning.

Clean storage areas should contain only clean material, and sharps containers should be routinely replaced when full. Nothing looks worse to a surveyor than seeing overflowing sharps containers, cluttered hallways, and equipment overdue for preventative maintenance.

The OR should have accurate humidity control, be clean and be in good repair. Expect the surveyors to inspect the OR, usually during off-hours. If your staff present a surgical suite as "ready" for the next patient, then it will be expected to meet all the requirements. Stained floors or equipment will result in citation.

If your biomedical equipment maintenance is performed under contract, make sure that your facilities staff are on top of this, and that the maintenance is completed on the specifications established by the manufacturer. Any reports to FDA on equipment malfunctions must be provided to surveyors upon request.

Finally, there is ample material in the Physical Environment and Fire Safety CoPs to establish a set of effective indicators for the facility's QAPI program. The focus should be on both patient and employee safety in the patient care environment.

482.42 Condition of Participation: Infection Control

The requirements of this CoP are stringent, and in these days of antibiotic-resistant organisms, and the threat of bioterrorism, they lend themselves to special consideration. As mentioned previously with the QAPI CoP, infection control tends to be a target of cost-cutting through its assignment to staff who have other responsibilities as well. Be careful not to take this Condition too lightly. Merely reviewing the infection rate monthly and reviewing the latest CDC information does not constitute an infection-control program. Surveyors will be looking for this program to be interwoven with your medical staff's patient-care peer review, nursing, P&T, facilities management, and laboratory, to name a few. Like QAPI, this program needs to be integrated to ensure its effectiveness. There will be one surveyor, probably a registered nurse, who will be designated to review compliance with this CoP.

Your facility should have a clear organizational chart showing who is responsible as infection-control officer. There is no definition for the qualifications of the infection-control officer, and, as noted, it may be more than one person. Typically, surveyors will see a hospital with a registered nurse and medical staff member designated as the infection-control officers. However they may be designated, the process must be effective. Any medical-staff physician so designated will be expected to perform this role.

As set forth in the standard for responsibilities, the CEO, medical staff, and director of nursing all are responsible for the implementation and effectiveness of this program. The infection-control program is a key component in the hospitalwide QAPI program. The surveyor will expect to see an active program in place.

482.43 Condition of Participation: Discharge Planning

This CoP sets forth the expectations for the discharge-planning process. This is a vulnerable area for hospital compliance, particularly since patients being prepared for discharge will undoubtedly find themselves being interviewed by the surveyors.

The evaluation process should start at admission, and should be the responsibility of a registered nurse, social worker, or "qualified individual" as described in the CoP. It is reasonable to expect that surveyors will interview patients who may need posthospital care. The IGs lay out the process for evaluation. It will be very embarrassing, and potentially problematic for the hospital, if a poststroke patient is described as ready for discharge, but has a hospital-acquired decubitus ulcer, no speech-therapy evaluation (if needed), and is targeted for home care without necessary support services. Hospitals are under tremendous pressure to move patients out of the acute area. A patient who has been properly prepared will result in fewer complaints and a better relationship with your post-hospital care providers. This, in turn, lessens the possibility of complaints finding their way to CMS and a compliance investigator appearing at your door.

As mentioned previously, your facility should be able to identify *all* posthospital care providers for a patient needing such care. Do not list only your own facility's posthospital care providers. The IGs give clear guidance for how a hospital may find a list of long-term-care skilled nursing facilities.

Don't give your discharge-planning staff additional responsibilities. As you evaluate the requirements of this CoP, there is much detail that goes into a successful discharge-planning program. It must also have its own QAPI program, especially to determine if the discharge-planning program in the hospital is up to date and effective.

482.44 Condition of Participation: Organ Procurement Responsibilities.

This Condition was created several years ago, following a dismal record of organ donation and procurement in this country. The focal point has become the hospitals, and in some states legislation is currently in existence to encourage the procurement process—more so than the actual donation. As in the case of CoPs where there is new or greater emphasis, the IGs lay out the expectations clearly. An individual in the hospital or the organ procurement organization (OPO) should coordinate the evaluation process. A formal agreement must be in place with the local OPO, and a means of coordinating procurement. Your facility must cooperate with the local OPO to make this work. If for some reason the OPO is not cooperative, hospitals should not assume this to be a reason not to comply with these requirements. The standards give hospitals leeway to establish their own staff, when properly trained, to act as a requestor for organ donation. If the OPO does not have the resources to send a staff member into a hospital to act as a requestor, then the hospital must do so consistent with the requirements.

The next component of the CoP addresses hospitals that perform organ transplantation. CMS proposes to establish distinct CoPs for hospitals wishing to receive Medicare coverage for transplant surgeries. If your facility provides these services, you should check the *Federal Register* for any notice of impending intent to establish regulations in this area.

482.51 Condition of Participation: Surgical Services

Surgical services are identified as an optional service for an acute-care hospital. When such services are offered, whether inpatient or outpatient, it is expected that the hospital will comply. The requirements set forth in the staffing section, as well as who may be qualified to participate in surgical procedures, should be carefully reviewed. Make sure your staff members have appropriate credentials, consistent with state laws, and beware of any "outside" individuals being present during procedures. This would include a physician's first assistants, medical-equipment salespersons, or other observers who are present without being credentialed, or who do not have the patient's permission. Remember that the patient is the individual who grants consent, not the hospital or physician.

The balance of the IGs for this Condition are self-explanatory. Make sure consents are properly dated and timed, that they include all procedures proposed, and that the risks and benefits have been clearly explained.

An effective QAPI program should highlight hospital staff issues, involvement of the medical staff through surgical case review, and infection control.

482.52 Condition of Participation: Anesthesia Services

Like the surgical services CoP, this CoP is self-explanatory. If your facility uses certified registered nurse anesthetists, make sure you check with your state licensing agency to determine if the MD/DO supervision requirements pertain.

Anyone providing anesthesia is required to be properly trained and credentialed, including any staff administering monitored anesthesia care in diagnostic areas. Your anesthesiologists should be able to provide the credentials that staff should possess in order to administer anesthesia.

Note especially the pre- and postoperative anesthesia evaluation requirements. For some reason, these seem to be cited on surveys. Staff should ensure that evaluations are complete and signed with the content and in the time frames specified.

482.53 Condition of Participation: Nuclear Medicine Services

Like the Radiology CoP, this is self-explanatory as to the guidelines. Both the technical and professional components should have QAPI programs. The director of the service must be appropriately qualified and credentialed. Safety of staff and proper handling and disposal of radioactive material is also to be emphasized. The IGs point out common-sense requirements, and my earlier comments about radiology apply as well.

482.54 Condition of Participation: Outpatient Services

This CoP traditionally was not significantly emphasized, but has grown more relevant in recent years. The CoP mandates that any hospital providing outpatient services must "comply with the hospital CoPs," meaning that elements such as patients' rights, staffing, and medical records all apply to a hospital-based or sponsored clinic. Once again, the rule of thumb used by CMS is, "Who bills for the service?" If the service is billed to Medicare using the Medicare hospital reimbursement rate, then it is considered a hospital service. This holds true even if physicians provide services in a private-practice style, but are actually under the hospital's aegis. As we have emphasized throughout this book, if it is a hospital service, it must be organized and directed like a hospital service. There must be an individual accountable in the hospital administrative structure for the outpatient service, and he or she must oversee the service to provide adequate staffing and resources commensurate with the level of services provided.

482.55 Condition of Participation: Emergency Services

This CoP is rather brief, considering the impact emergency services has on a hospital's operation. Much of the emphasis on care has fallen into the EMTALA arena in recent years. However, the physician oversight of the service is important to the extent that the director is properly qualified, and that an effective QAPI program encompassing both the medical and professional staff is in place. Note the comment in the IGs relative to timeliness of support services being provided to patients (e.g., lab, radiology, etc.). Although these may not fall under EMTALA standards because the patient is in the hospital, a lack of timely diagnosis and treatment could lead to significant deficiencies if found during record review or patient interview.

Of particular interest is the mention again of having sufficient resources (in this case, staffing) in the event of disaster. It should be realized that disaster preparation is a key component of hospital services nowadays, and will probably receive more attention as events proceed.

482.56 Condition of Participation: Rehabilitation Services

When a hospital provides speech, audiology, occupational, or physical therapy, these services fall under this CoP. These services may be provided individually, or in combination with the other services shown above. Note that the CoP does not include cardiac rehabilitation as part of rehab services.

The rehab service needs to be directed by a properly qualified individual. The CoP does not mandate that a single person be director of all services if multiple services are provided.

Qualifications of staff and the policies and procedures of the service(s) must also be approved by the medical staff. Surveyors should be easily able to locate for review evidence of a signoff by the medical staff.

482.57 Condition of Participation: Respiratory Services

As with the previous CoPs, this is straightforward and does not require additional detail. It is important to comment here regarding the provision of services by staff other than respiratory therapists. In some cases, properly trained RNs have been allowed to provide these services. Both a qualified respiratory therapist and the medical staff should review this. You should also ensure that your facility does not run afoul of state licensure or limits of practice when assigning respiratory-therapy duties to anyone other than respiratory therapists.

CHAPTER 4

Know your role
on survey day

Know your role on survey day

Now that we've covered the CoPs, here are some tips for survey day:

Accompany the surveyors if at all possible, and watch what they see, hear, and do.

Never leave surveyors to their own devices or on their own in your facility unless they specifically request it. As they progress to each department or service, someone should anticipate their arrival and be there to greet them. That person should be a point person for that department. Remember, surveys are unannounced and can occur when your department heads are on vacation. Backup staff should be designated beforehand in the event this happens. Unit nursing directors can be excellent persons to use as backups when the nursing director is on vacation. When backup staff is unavailable, it may fall upon the survey coordinator to cover for that service or department. I don't recommend this, as it ties up the coordinator in dealing with a specific area and may prevent him or her from seeing the broader picture of the survey from the perspective of the surveyors.

Surveyors will definitely want to have time alone to discuss their findings and arrange for completion of the survey process. Respect their need by providing a single location for them to meet, along with a phone for contact purposes. Always have a list of staff members they can contact in each department or service, and don't hesitate to contact those staff members on your own if necessary.

You might be able to prep the staff before the surveyors arrive, because as survey coordinator you should have an idea of where the survey is heading, and how the information from all the departments and services affected may be turning into deficiencies.

Watch what is happening in each area every day the survey continues. Listen to the questions and answers between surveyors and staff. They may tell you something about what the surveyor is looking for, or where deficiencies may lie. In an allegation survey, this may give you an idea of the complaint or problem that was reported to CMS, and accordingly help you develop a response.

This also goes to what I mentioned in the introduction: you can control the survey by expediting what the surveyors need and by clearing the process of any obstructions. Department head can't come in? Arrange a teleconference. Can't find a document? Put someone else on the hunt, and get back to ensuring the survey continues without interruption, or your presence.

Intercede to prevent misunderstandings. Communicate frequently with the surveyor or survey team.

It is important that the survey coordinator understand what is happening on each service or department as the survey progresses. Since the survey coordinator is usually one person, it becomes critical for the point person in each service or department to respond to the surveyors when they need answers or assistance, and that the information communicated is summarized to the survey coordinator. If something is stated incorrectly, make sure you contact the surveyors to correct the misunderstanding. In addition, ask for periodic updates from the survey staff, although they may wish to provide such information only at the exit conference.

In any event, even if you only ask the surveyors, "How are you doing and do you need anything?" that may be the most important action of the entire survey. You should check with them at least twice a day, unless they direct you otherwise. Keep the process moving and you could see the survey completed in the least amount of time necessary or desired.

Even if the survey appears to be going badly, learn to develop positive, action-based responses. Although it may not affect the outcome, it will mitigate future problems.

Always start corrective action the minute you know a surveyor has detected a problem. They may not tell you if it is a deficiency or not, but if they mention it, you can bet it is at least of concern to them. Also, knowing the CoPs will help you know if a deficiency is being identified or not.

If a problem is identified, don't play the blame game. Have the department or service head develop and implement corrective action. It will bring you into compliance, and it will look great on your corrective action plan to CMS if you initiate corrective action the day the deficiency is identified. It certainly makes executing your plan of correction a whole lot easier.

Know what to do next

Know what to do next

Once the surveyor or survey team lets you know it is finished, you should specifically request an exit conference, unless you have done so earlier. Surveyors are required to offer you the opportunity for an exit, so make sure you take it. Let's cover what to do:

1. Preparation for the exit conference

Gather all the survey status reports you have accumulated over the course of the survey. That may be just one day, and if so, make sure you bring in all the staff members who were subject to the survey for discussion on what was covered by the surveyors, what potential issues were found or perceived, and any corrective action implemented or being developed.

2. Limit participation

Although it is good to have staff members present to hear the surveyors, you don't want to intimidate them by having everyone present who happens to be in the hospital. I have attended exit interviews in large amphitheaters, and watched staff joking around and asking, "Why are we here?" Well, they didn't need to be there. It also has a tendency to intimidate the surveyors, which I can assure you is not good. Only key department heads or staff should be present, and the meeting should take place in a room conducive to discussion. Don't pick a large auditorium or amphitheater.

Some tips for the exit conference:

- At least initially, I do not suggest the presence of hospital counsel unless you or your staff members have received some indication of a significant problem. The findings presented in the exit conference are preliminary. Only the Statement of Deficiencies (CMS 2567) report, when issued, is the final summary of survey findings. Some counsels may be eager to contest findings and could inadvertently start an adversarial relationship with the survey team. This can put surveyors on the defensive, and inhibit the possibility of discussion between the hospital and surveyors at the time of the exit as to their findings.

• If you decide to videotape or audiotape the exit conference, you will be required to provide an additional audio or videotape recorder to survey staff to record the exit interview as well.

• The exit conference is the presentation of findings from the survey. Some survey teams may be able to issue their findings via computer system during the exit interview. At some time during the survey, you should ask if the survey team will be issuing a CMS 2567 at the exit interview. In this case, if it makes you feel more comfortable, you could then have counsel present. It is purely an option on the part of the provider being surveyed. Counsel was rarely present at any exit conference I participated in.

• It is always best to maintain a professional and open attitude during the exit conference. If you are unclear on any findings, you should ask the surveyor to clarify. If it appears that a surveyor may have missed an important piece of information, mention it and have staff immediately find that information for presentation to the surveyor. A deficiency corrected during the survey will probably still be cited. The surveyor may add a comment that it was corrected during the survey. However, the fact that a surveyor and not your staff identified it is a question to be asked through your QAPI process, and you may have to present that as a plan of correction.

• Do not get into heated arguments with the surveyors. It will not accomplish anything other than to hamper a relationship you will have with the survey team after the survey is concluded. You can state your disagreement, and then wait to see what will be issued. You will then have an opportunity to review what is cited, and also review the IGs in this book, as well as the regulation itself.

The Statement of Deficiencies

The method of communicating the findings from any CMS survey is via the Statement of Deficiencies and Provider Plan of Correction. There are no "positives" reported in the 2567, only deficiencies found. If no deficiencies were identified, you will still receive a 2567 form, but do not be alarmed. There should be a statement to the effect that the "facility was in compliance with program requirements" or "found in compliance with 42 *CFR XXXX*."

The 2567 is generated using a computer software package called ASPEN. The system will first automatically print out, word for word, the Condition, standard, or element being cited. It may be alarming when you receive a 2567 report, because there may be numerous pages to it. Again, this may be because the deficiency being cited is attached to a lengthy regulation, and at the end the surveyors will provide the reason for the citation. The actual deficiency starts at that point.

As a reference, the system prints a tag number next to each deficiency (e.g., A071). This tag number can help locate the area being cited much more easily than reference to the legal regulation number. It will also help you locate the CoP where the citation exists. Refer to the CoPs provided in this book and you will be able to refer to the citations with ease via the tag number.

Surveyors have been instructed at length about the verbiage they should use in a Statement of Deficiencies. Words such as "inappropriately" and "unacceptable" are not to be used by surveyors unless there is sufficient description of what was unacceptable or inappropriate. Surveyors are also to be as specific as possible when identifying a deficiency, and should refer to specific patients or medical records. This will usually be done with a unique identifier assigned to that record by the surveyor. You will be provided with a key sheet to identify the patient record. If you are unable to identify the patient record, or the citation is not clear, you should contact the survey agency before submitting your plan of correction (POC).

You should receive the Statement of Deficiencies not more than two weeks after the survey. In the cover transmittal letter, you will be instructed as to where to submit your plan of correction, and when it is due. In the intervening time between the exit conference and the receipt of the Statement of Deficiencies, you should have started to assign your key staff members with the initiation of a corrective action plan. You may only have two weeks to submit a corrective action plan after receipt of the Statement of Deficiencies, so time is at a premium. There are more stringent time frames when CoPs are determined to be out of compliance, which we will cover further on.

The Plan of Correction

Once a Statement of Deficiencies is issued, it becomes the official report of the survey conducted in your facility. It is also a public document, subject to release to requesting parties under the Freedom of Information Law. The facility's plan of correction, when submitted and approved by CMS, also becomes a matter of public record. Only patient or staff identifiers are prohibited from release. Accordingly, it behooves a facility to put a good plan of correction into writing. We will discuss the format for writing a plan of correction, and what and what not to say.

Specificity

The main thrust of any POC should be to directly address the citation. Do not attempt to write lengthy defenses of your facility's care, or put your mission statement in the POC. It will not help your cause. Each POC should identify how the deficiency will be corrected and who will be responsible for ensuring the corrective action is monitored and completed. Finally, and most important, a completion date for the corrective action will be necessary. Do not put "ongoing" or "completed" next to a POC in the area marked for completion on the Statement of Deficiencies. Make sure you respond to every deficiency, even those that only cross reference another citation. In other words, you may see a deficiency under the Governing Body CoP with cross-reference to a citation under the QAPI CoP. Remember that there is interconnection between CoPs, so you should examine what the surveyors are telling you. In the case mentioned, a response might be to indicate how the Governing Body will ensure correction of the QAPI deficiency.

Refutation and errors

There will be occasions on which you discover there is an error in the Statement of Deficiencies issued by the survey team. Contact the surveyors to inform them. You must submit any information substantiating the error. For example, if an H&P was cited for being missing but was part of the record during the survey, you should send the document to the surveyors as part of the POC. Do not redact patient information, as it will make it impossible to identify the record. In the POC, use language such as, "We respectfully wish to point out that the record . . . etc." It is definitely unacceptable to insert corrections into records or other documents after the citations identify them, and then submit this to the surveyors as an error on their part.

Refutation is often the element that can cause the most headaches for both parties involved. It usually is an emotional response on the part of the facility to the citations, and tends to sound overly defensive (and in some cases, offensive) to surveyors. You may firmly believe that the surveyor has a grudge, doesn't like you or your staff, or is incompetent. An objective review of your Statement of Deficiencies will probably show some, if not all, truth to the citations. Imagine what a newspaper could do with an overly defensive POC. Nobody will benefit from an emotionally charged response. Keep your emotions in check and your POC will reflect a professional and objective approach.

Major problems following a survey

As a Medicare provider, your facility must undergo some form of periodic inspection. When you fail to prepare for it, it can bring down the wrath of CMS and threaten your continued participation in the Medicare (and Medicaid, for reasons previously stated) program. When the survey is concluded, surveyors will tally up their information and present it in the 2567 report. If the deficiencies found are significant enough, CMS may instruct surveyors to issue a noncompliance decision with one or more of the CoPs. This can be based upon:

- Immediate jeopardy to the health of patients or a patient

- Inability to effectively deliver services in accordance with the standard of care

- Significant or dangerous fire-safety or environmental issues

Further on, we will discuss in greater detail more serious deficiencies which invoke the term "Immediate Jeopardy."

Whenever Conditions are cited as noncompliant as a result of a survey, the facility is immediately placed on a termination track. This notice is usually issued either directly by CMS or through the survey team after CMS has reviewed the findings. Under no circumstances do the surveyors make such a determination without consulting CMS.

When Conditions are not in compliance

Any Medicare provider must take special and immediate notice when a CoP is determined out of compliance. Continued participation in the Medicare program is automatically put on a termination track when this occurs. If the deficiencies leading to the CoP being determined noncompliant are not corrected, then termination takes effect. Although there is an appellate process for termination proceedings, do you really want to go through all the aggravation? Your facility will still have to correct the deficiencies cited.

Most importantly, a good POC will put your facility in better stead with the federal government. The memory of a poor outcome on a survey exists for a long time after the survey is done, especially with the surveyors, who you may see again.

There are two types of Condition-level deficiency status that enter in here. The following is the process which is followed in two types of situations where Condition-level noncompliance is identified as a result of the survey:

Serious and imminent threat Condition non compliance:

- First is the most serious, where the deficiencies demonstrate a serious and imminent threat to patient safety. These can be of a quality-of-care or LSC nature. You should receive these deficiencies within two days of the last day of the survey. These deficiencies will cause the facility to be terminated from Medicare within 23 days after the last day of the survey unless the deficiencies in the CoP(s) cited are corrected. The term "corrected" does not mean that a POC about the deficiencies is submitted and approved, though that will still be required in the time frames stipulated when the deficiencies are transmitted to the facility.

- The CoP deficiencies that are out of compliance must also be substantially corrected within the 23-day period. If Condition-level noncompliance is identified, it is strongly suggested that an ad hoc committee or team be formed to ensure correction within the 23 days. These are calendar days, not business days. The surveyors who conducted the initial survey and identified the CoP as noncompliant may return to the facility to determine if the deficiencies for that CoP have been corrected. This will only be done if the facility requests it in writing, and in that communication indicates that the deficiencies are corrected.

- A resurvey of that CoP's deficiencies must take place, and the facility must be found to have corrected the deficiencies for termination proceedings to be stopped. There are no extensions of this timetable, so ensure that you take corrective action within the timeframes stipulated.

- The state agency surveyors, upon determination that the deficiencies are corrected, will recommend that CMS stop termination proceedings. The decision is left to CMS. If your facility has had a pattern of noncompliance over a period of time, CMS could decide to maintain the termination proceedings. If so, you should then contact CMS and contact your counsel.

Limited-capacity Condition noncompliance

This is a less serious form of Condition-level deficiencies, but they must be taken as seriously as those noted above. The same circumstances apply (i.e., termination from Medicare) but the time period to correct deficiencies is extended to 45 days from the last day of the survey. All other requirements apply as noted above, including the need to actually correct the deficiencies cited, and have a resurvey for the CoP deficiencies before the end of the 45 days.

As a final note:

- Remember that the state survey agency and CMS must first approve any corrective action before you initiate it. The state agency will consult with CMS so you should not have to do both. In some cases, your corrective action plan may go directly to CMS, and approval of it will be issued from them.

- Do not issue a corrective action plan without full intent to correct the deficiencies. Your facility's reputation with Medicare rests with your sincerity in correcting the problems.

- Whenever there are disagreements, work first with your state agency unless the deficiencies were issued directly from CMS. The government tries to keep facilities in the Medicare program if they show effective corrective action. Always try to negotiate if you have concerns or if you have problems implementing a plan of correction after it has been approved.

Immediate jeopardy

This term originated from the long-term-care side of CMS. It was intended to identify serious deficiencies that threaten patients' well being. We have appended a copy of the guidance provided to CMS surveyors for immediate jeopardy. It most often is applied when actual patient harm or the potential for harm is observed. Since CMS hospital surveyors now conduct patient interviews on the care units in the hospital, there is obviously more opportunity to identify problems.

Immediate jeopardy citations follow the 23-day termination track. There may be significant deficiencies to correct, such as retraining staff, implementing sweeping changes in procedures, or having to get all the medical staff to approve new policies and implement them. All this would have to be accomplished in the 23-day period.

Know how to respond

Know how to respond

After the exit conference is over and the surveyors are gone, it is often thought that the worst is over. Not to burst the proverbial bubble, but the next step is the most important and can be the most troublesome. Although you may have had an exit conference, the only official report from a CMS survey is contained on the CMS 2567 form. It is on this form that you will find any deficiencies noted during the survey and the corresponding requirement for the particular Condition, standard, or element will be stated just prior to the actual deficiency. In fact, if no deficiencies are found on a survey, CMS will require the CMS 2567 form to be sent to the hospital with a statement to the effect that the facility is "in substantial compliance with program requirements." Yes, there are occasions when that actually happens.

However, more often than not, there will be a deficiency or deficiencies identified. It usually falls to the survey coordinator to compile the POC, and perhaps actually prepare the written response. This is a job that may seem relatively innocuous, but is filled with pitfalls. The other problem is that some proficiency in developing positive responses is needed. One does not have to be a literary genius, but it helps to understand how to use the right words and phrases.

In a Joint Commission–accredited hospital, this may be the first occasion that a POC will have to be prepared. Use the following tips to prepare a successful response:

- Typically, you will have approximately 10–15 calendar days to respond to a Statement of Deficiencies (the time varies based sometimes on mailing time and severity of the deficiencies cited). This must be a written plan outlining how the facility will correct deficiencies, and monitor their correction. Some of the deficiencies will be minor, some significant. The levels of deficiencies start at the element level (individual components of a standard), progress to standard level (a compilation of elements), then to a Condition level (a compilation of standards and elements). The surveyor determines deficiencies based on factual information in the record, observations, and sometimes clinical or professional judgment.

- One person should gather all the responses. The actual response should come in some form from each affected department or service. However, one person should take responsibility for ensuring that the entire corrective action plan is consistent, covers the basic requirements of the POC, and avoids any potential problems in interpretation.

- Do not delay meeting the CMS timetable. If a POC action needs more development, you may respond that "Quality Improvement and the department head will meet on [insert specific date] to implement the first steps of corrective action as follows," and then list specific first steps to correct the problem. For example, if a policy or procedure needs modification, indicate that it will be changed following development of a "best practice" for the facility. However, do not leave it at that. Make sure the problem that caused the deficiency is eliminated by taking immediate action that will at least mitigate the problem until the full fix is implemented.

- As noted above, don't be afraid to "stage" your POC. Indicate the timetable with a series of milestone dates for ultimate correction. For example, if a number of patients were found with decubiti on a given floor of the hospital, and this was cited as poor nursing care, a corrective action plan could involve monitoring on an ongoing basis, development of new training to prevent decubiti, and formation of skin-care teams, as one possible plan. Each will require a specific amount of time to accomplish.

- Do not ask for an extension to submit your plan. It will probably not be approved anyway, and it can imply that you may not be taking the survey seriously, or don't understand how to comply with the CoPs.

Know the ambulatory surgery center survey

Know the ambulatory surgery center survey

Many ambulatory surgery centers (ASC) do not have the luxury of a distinct survey coordinator who does not manage any clinical components. Often, the surgical nurse director wears many hats, and is sometimes required to deal with surveyors. However, the administrator of the ASC will often coordinate at least the nonclinical portions of the survey. Surveys can put a strain on the operations of the facility if there is not sufficient care taken to be ready for any type of surveillance by CMS. As with hospital surveys, the ASC survey is unannounced. You may have your busiest day of surgery when this happens, so be prepared. You cannot ask the surveyors to come back later when you aren't so busy.

I will not cover in detail any tips for ASC surveillance, because most of what applies to hospitals applies as well to ASCs. Of course, there is a more limited scale, but nonetheless CMS expects more from ASCs because they have grown in scope and complexity.

CMS is proposing several changes/additions to the ASC CoPs at this time. Here's a look at the proposed changes and how they will affect ASCs:

Governance (Sec. 416.41)

This would give additional duties to the governing body of the ASC. This may be the physician ownership of the ASC, or any other individuals who are part of the ASC governance. Note that the changes mandate oversight of the facility QAPI program. This oversight must be reflected in the meetings of the governing authority, as a specific topic in minutes with findings, conclusions, and recommendations for the program's outcomes. In some ASCs in which low-risk procedures are performed, this may be glossed over.

The governing body should be cognizant of its need to "dig deeper" if the program continues to report the same information month after month with no change.

The governing body also has to ensure that all policies and procedures promote patient health and safety, and that the facility develops and implements an effective disaster plan. The latter element, which is new to ASCs, grows out of our need to be more prepared for the many disasters that can and have befallen us. The disaster plan must be tailored to the individual region in which the ASC operates. Because the ASC relies more on a scheduled day and is not subject to 24/7 operation and emergency response, there certainly is less about which to be concerned. However, the governing body must ensure that its patients are in the highest state of safety and security. Lastly, ASC directors should watch very carefully for the Interpretive Guidelines that will follow this change if it is approved and becomes a regulation. Your governing-body minutes will have to cover much more in the areas of quality of care, operation, and patient safety. Fortunately, many ASCs possess some form of accreditation, so this and the other changes to the CoPs will simply mirror current accreditation requirements.

Sec. 416.43 Conditions for coverage—Quality assessment and performance improvement.

I will not belabor what is mandated in this revised CoP, other than to say that the data-driven approach means more data collection and analysis. It is not acceptable merely to report that X number of procedures were performed and no problems were identified. In an ASC in which low-risk procedures are performed, this may be the case, but there is always room for analysis. In an eye surgery center, it may benefit the QAPI program to look at the FMEA approach for assessing risk. Simply put, this process analyzes the extent to which a system will continue to use a specific format until it breaks. Knowing where the breaking point is and what causes that breakage marks successful implementation of this process. Incidents occur in these settings, such as wrong lens/wrong patient, or error in or diversion from accepted technique. Using FMEA, are there any points during the entire process of patient booking to patient discharge and follow-up that have the potential for problems? How often are these opportunities for problems occurring? Have there been "near misses," and have those been reviewed by staff members to determine their significance? Is your infection-control program part of this assessment process? All these elements play into the governing authority's responsibility to ensure the health and safety of its patients. It will not be acceptable to simply report numbers month after month without truly analyzing them.

Sec. 416.50 Conditions for coverage—Patients' rights

This new CoP may seem innocuous at first, but note that among other things it requires disclosure of physician ownership or financial interest in the ASC to the patient. The patient has to be given information that he or she can understand that clearly delineates his or her rights, the ability to file a grievance if a patient so desires, and the process that is used to resolve the grievance. Note as well the need to provide patients with advance-directive information as to how the ASC will allow those directives to be implemented. This certainly calls for recognition of advance directives, and policies and procedures to handle these in the event they must be utilized.

There are also reporting requirements for certain violations of a patient's physical well-being, including following state reporting laws where required. Make sure you are aware of any reporting (including to local law enforcement agencies) for any violations that could necessitate contact with outside authorities.

Finally, be careful about the competency issues mentioned at the end of the CoP. The courts or other legal means are typically used to establish competence. It is going to be very important that an ASC ensure that competency rulings are followed when dealing with certain types or classes of patients.

Sec. 416.51 Conditions for coverage—Infection Control

Not much needs to be said about this CoP, other than that it follows a similar format to the hospital CoP as far as integration of findings into QAPI, and the designation of a specific qualified person to be responsible for the infection-control program. Be careful to ensure that the program covers all aspects of the center's operation, not only from the clinical side, but the general environmental side as well.

Sec. 416.52 Conditions for coverage—Patient admission, assessment and discharge

This last new CoP is very interesting. In this set of proposed changes, the regulations limit stays in an ASC up to 11:59 p.m. the day of the surgical procedure. That may not be too problematic for most ASCs but the last element of this CoP raises some questions. It stipulates that "each patient has a discharge order, signed by a physician or the qualified practitioner who performed the surgery or procedure unless otherwise specified by state law. The discharge order must indicate that the patient has been evaluated for proper anesthesia and medical recovery."

At what point must the patient be evaluated, and by whom? If physicians leave as soon as the procedure is done, and the procedure appears to be successful, yet the patient is still recovering from the procedure, who will evaluate the patient for recovery for medical and anesthesia purposes? If the patient has a slow or difficult recovery, how will that be handled with reference to this CoP? Watch this carefully, because these regulations were still in the comment stage as of this writing.

Know how to select a survey coordinator

Know how to select
a survey coordinator

This chapter is aimed at CEOs and other health leaders.

In my 30-plus years of performing acute-care, ambulatory-surgery, and outpatient surveys for CMS in my state agency, I could always tell who was "on the ball" when we arrived on site. A good survey coordinator is worth his or her weight in gold. I have seen CEOs, vice presidents, and others try to perform this function while trying to keep up with the business of the facility. That can be a real trap, often resulting in a poor survey outcome.

Here are some "do's and don'ts" for selecting a survey coordinator:

- DO pick a qualified staff member, generally recommended to be a person with clinical background. Your medical director may have his or her feathers ruffled, but he or she should stick to medical-staff issues and not try to coordinate the survey. Often, the quality improvement coordinator, who is usually a nurse by background, ends up being the survey coordinator. He or she may have the broadest knowledge of the hospital operation through dealing with department heads and coordinating medical-staff issues with the medical-staff leadership.

- DON'T try to write the plan of correction by yourself, fail to involve the department heads and staff members involved, or make the survey coordinator write the plan alone. I recall a CEO who used to write the plan of correction for a CMS full survey of his hospital. One time, he failed to tell the department heads and staff what he told CMS they would do to correct the problems. The hospital came to the brink of Medicare and Medicaid decertification. Everyone in the facility should know how to develop an effective plan of correction. Holding an inservice using some of the tips in this book will help in that regard.

- DO give authority to the survey coordinator to deal with problems that arise during a survey. Let department heads know that they have the authority to issue orders if necessary, and to correct problems immediately if the surveyors find deficiencies. Again, there is a trust and competence issue here. That's why a good survey coordinator is so valuable.

- DON'T overrule your survey coordinator if the surveyors find problems and they recommend immediate correction. The survey coordinator should have a keen sense of how the survey is progressing. He or she may see a major problem that might be mitigated by immediate correction.

- DO communicate routinely with the survey coordinator during the survey and afterwards until the plan of correction is accepted by CMS or the state survey agency. He or she will be able to help you plan for your responses, and more importantly, will let you know where there are problems that surveyors have found.

CHAPTER 9

Presurvey checklist for CoP compliance

Presurvey checklist for CoP compliance

The purpose of this checklist is to give hospital staff a "quick read" of the highlights of each Centers for Medicare & Medicare Services' (CMS) Condition of Participation (CoP) for hospitals. It is not intended to replace the text of this book as far as the individual guidance for each CoP. Each CoP and Interpretive Guideline should be fully reviewed to ensure compliance.

Governing body:

❑ Quality assurance performance improvement (QAPI) plan and program in place.

❑ Data collection and analysis methods for QAPI approved by governing body.

❑ Governing body minutes show evidence of QAPI oversight.

❑ New medical staff appropriately approved by governing body.

❑ Medical Staff recredentialing completed in accord with medical staff and governing body bylaws.

❑ All contracts current and reflected in QAPI program.

❑ Infection control program in place and reporting through the QAPI program.

❑ Indicators developed for evaluating and assuring patient safety.

❑ Three year capital budget and current operating budget developed and approved by governing body.

❑ Clear process established to oversight implementation of Patients' Rights provisions.

❑ Medical Staff Bylaws, rules and regulations, and /or policies and procedures are current and address regulatory requirements.

❑ Verbal order policy allows flexibility within scope of CMS rules, but ensures patient safety.

Patients' rights:

    ❑ Written patients' rights handout developed for distribution to patients.

    ❑ Patient grievance policy in place.

    ❑ All complaints to hospital show evidence of investigation and response.

    ❑ Staff are knowledgeable of existence of grievance policy and process.

    ❑ Advance directives honored in accord with patients' wishes and state laws.

    ❑ Restraint policy in place, approved and implemented by both medical staff and nursing.

    ❑ Any patient deaths occurring while the patient was in restraint or seclusion have been reported to CMS.

    ❑ Pain management policy and procedure developed and implemented. The policy should involve the patient in the pain management decision-making process.

    ❑ Restraints should always be the least restrictive, and follow strict review protocols before implementation.

QAPI:

    ❑ QAPI plan approved and in place, and QAPI staff oversight evident.

    ❑ All QAPI reports from medical staff and hospital departments current and approved.

    ❑ Indicators for high-risk and problem-prone areas reviewed for each department and service.

    ❑ Adverse events have been fully reviewed, causes found and corrective action taken.

    ❑ Specific quality improvement projects identified and processed.

    ❑ Statistical and objective data from each area subject to QAPI review is gathered, analyzed and becomes a routine reporting element of the QAPI program.

Medical staff:

    ❑ All physicians and licensed independent practitioners (LIP) currently licensed and registered as required.

    ❑ Files contain evidence of primary source verification of licensure and National Practitioner Data Bank inquiry.

❏ Files contain evidence of appointment to leadership positions:

  – Medical director

  – Emergency services

  – Radiology

  – Nuclear medicine

  – Laboratory/pathology

  – Respiratory services

  – Critical care

  – Anesthesia services

Bylaws current and descriptive of medical staff organization.

Nursing services:

❏ Director of nursing identified and qualified.

❏ All staff possess current licensure, registration, or certification as needed. Files contain primary source verification.

❏ Evidence of RN supervision and oversight of care.

❏ Medication administration completed in accord with professional principles and state laws.

❏ Evidence of collaboration between pharmacist and nursing staff to develop polices and procedures.

❏ Verbal orders used infrequently by medical staff or LIPs.

❏ Transfusion reactions reported in accordance with developed policy. Corrective action implemented when necessary.

Medical record services:

❏ Staff qualified and sufficient for the size and complexity of the hospital.

❏ Records files are easily retrievable.

❏ Process followed for ensuring staff compliance with record completeness.

❏ Confidentiality maintained for all records.

❑ Polices and procedures followed for release of medical records to patients and other parties.

❑ History and physical (H&P) exams completed on a timely basis.

❑ HIPAA notification to all patients in place and documented.

Pharmacy services:

❑ Services directed by a pharmacist or consulting pharmacist.

❑ Drug storage safely maintained in accord with federal and state laws.

❑ Drugs and biologicals kept in locked storage/refrigerated as required.

❑ Adverse drug reactions evaluated.

❑ All drugs and biologicals are not beyond expiration dates.

❑ Losses and diversions of medications reported to appropriate authorities and QAPI program.

❑ Formulary in place and modified after approval of medical staff.

Radiological services:

❑ Staff properly licensed and qualified for their positions.

❑ Safety precautions identified in writing and followed by all staff.

❑ Equipment properly maintained and periodically tested.

❑ Films/records kept in accord with statutes or policy.

❑ All reports read by radiologists or practitioners who perform radiological services.

Laboratory services:

❑ All necessary CLIA certifications are present and current.

❑ Services are provided consistent with hospital size and complexity 24 hours a day.

❑ Any blood/blood products testing positive for HIV after previously testing negative must be quarantined, and any affected patients notified.

❑ Notification is made to attending physician, and either the attending or hospital makes patient notification, or notification to patient's responsible party as appropriate.

Food and dietetic services:

❏ Services must be directed by a qualified food service director.

❏ Services can be provided by an outside entity as long as a dietitian is retained by the hospital.

❏ The dietitian must be retained as employee or consultant to assess patient needs.

❏ Therapeutic dietary manual must be current and available for all medical nursing and food service staff.

❏ All patients requiring dietary intervention should have such done in accordance with standards of care.

Utilization review:

❏ If a hospital has an agreement with an approved quality improvement organization, this condition will not be surveyed by CMS.

❏ Otherwise, a utilization review (UR) plan and UR committee must review lengths of stay and make determinations of medical necessity for admission and length of stay.

Physical environment:

❏ All buildings must be maintained in accord with the National Fire Protection Association's *Life Safety Code® (LSC)* and principles of safe operation.

❏ Emergency lighting must be present in the OR, recovery room, intensive care, emergency service and all stairwells. Backup battery power for emergency lighting is also required.

❏ The year 2000 edition of the *LSC* must be met.

❏ Waivers from compliance with the *LSC* may be granted if unreasonable hardship can be shown, without adverse effect on patient safety.

❏ State provisions may overrule the *LSC* if it can be shown they are equal to or greater than the *LSC* provisions, and are approved by CMS.

❏ The hospital must have an effective disaster plan in the event of a disaster or emergency.

❏ Trash and hazardous waste must be disposed in an acceptable manner.

Infection control:

❑ There must be a designated infection control officer.

❑ A system for identification and management of infections must be in place.

❑ A system for evaluating the causes and scope of infections must be in place.

❑ A log must be in place to track all infections.

Discharge planning:

❑ All patients in need of discharge planning are identified.

❑ Each patient needing discharge planning has an evaluation completed to determine the extent of services needed.

❑ Family or responsible parties for patients should be involved in the planning process.

❑ Patients should be reassessed as needed.

Organ tissue and eye procurement:

❑ An agreement must exist between the hospital and the designated organ procurement agency.

❑ An agreement must also exist with at least one eye bank and one tissue bank. Every potential donor must be identified and the patient or responsible party interviewed as to the possibility of donation.

❑ There should be evidence of periodic educational sessions with staff and designated requestors to address procedures for organ donation requests.

❑ Facilities which perform organ transplants must be members of the Organ Procurement and Transplantation Network.

OPTIONAL SERVICES

Surgical services:

❑ The operating room must be supervised by an experienced MD, DO, or RN.

❑ Licensed practical nurses (LPN) and surgical techs may serve as scrub nurses in accord with state law and under the supervision of an RN.

❑ RNs may be circulating nurses; LPNs and surgical techs may assist when under the supervision of an RN and consistent with state laws.

❑ All H&Ps must be in patients' charts before surgery.

❑ Consents should be valid for the procedure(s) being planned.

❑ Operative reports should be in the record immediately following surgery.

Anesthesia services:

❑ Services must be directed by an individual qualified to perform anesthesia.

❑ Preanesthesia evaluations are to be performed not more than 48 hours prior to surgery.

❑ Postanesthesia follow-up must be documented within 48 hours after the procedure.

❑ Physician supervision of certified registered nurse anesthetists should be determined consistent with those states in which CMS has granted a waiver.

Nuclear medicine:

❑ The director and staff must be appropriately qualified for their roles

❑ All radioactive material should be stored and disposed in accord with safe practice and state and federal laws.

❑ There should be continuing assessment and preventative maintenance for nuclear medicine equipment.

❑ Reports of procedures must be maintained for at least five years.

Outpatient services:

❑ Services must be integrated with the hospital's inpatient services.

❑ There needs to be a staff member whose overall responsibility is this service.

Emergency services:

❑ The service must be directed by a qualified member of the medical staff.

❑ Services must be integrated with the other services provided by the hospital.

❏ Policies and procedures are a responsibility of the medical staff.

❏ An adequate number of staff must be present to address the emergency needs of patients.

Rehabilitation services:

❏ The services must be headed by a qualified individual who has the experience necessary to manage the services.

❏ Practitioner orders for rehabilitation services are to be included in the medical record, along with a written plan of treatment.

Respiratory care services:

❏ The service is to be directed by an MD or DO with appropriate experience, on either a part-time or full-time basis.

❏ The medical staff must designate the qualifications of staff who provide respiratory care services.

❏ Services are to be provided on the order of a physician or LIP as appropriate.

CASE STUDY

The scenario

On Friday, January 20, an elderly patient is admitted to your facility through the emergency department (ED). She fell while being transferred at a local nursing home, and the primary diagnosis is a fractured hip. She also has severe Alzheimer's, diabetes, other comorbidities, and is on a host of medications. Otherwise, she had been in reasonably good physical health. She has a do-not-resuscitate order and healthcare proxy indicating no extraordinary means of life support.

While in the ED, the patient is observed thrashing and screaming, and medication does not help. She is restrained using wrist and ankle restraints so that she will not roll off the gurney. The ED is extremely busy, and she is rapidly sent to the floor. She continues her screaming and thrashing while being transferred to a bed, and nurses reapply the restraints. She appears to calm down, and because she has no existing primary physician, she is assigned to house staff. She is also assigned to the on call orthopedist, who has called and is on his way.

The in-house physician stops at the nurses' station to get the chart, and talks to nursing staff about the patient's behavior while being transferred. The charge nurse and the physician go to the patient's room, where the patient is found unresponsive. The children of the patient, who were in the waiting area to see their mother, become very upset and vocal. They loudly shout that the hospital has killed their mother and threaten to call the media.

An article appears in the next day's local newspaper, stating that the patient died "mysteriously." The hospital's public relations staff are quoted as stating that the patient was very ill, and that the hospital shares in the loss suffered by the children of the patient. The children meet with the administrator, and all appears to be smoothed over.

One week later, state agency surveyors arrive unannounced, and indicate they are performing an allegation survey of the following CoPs:

- Governing Body

- Medical Staff

- Patients' Rights

- Nursing

- Quality Assurance and Performance Improvement (QAPI)

- Emergency Services

The surveyors are an administrator and two nurses. As survey coordinator, you are asked for a list of current and previous admissions, and the surveyors choose a sample. You note that the elderly patient who died last week is on the list. One nurse surveyor starts reviewing the closed records; the other proceeds to Emergency Services, and then is scheduled to go to the floor. The administrator asks for Medical Staff Bylaws, the QAPI plan, minutes and or reports of QAI for the departments and services being reviewed.

What are your next steps?

Ten days after the survey concludes, the final report is received. On the CMS 2567 Statement of Deficiencies, the facility is found to have "Not Met" the CoPs of Nursing, Patients' Rights, Quality Assurance and Performance Improvement, and Governing Body. Other deficiencies are cited in the other CoPs but they are shown to be "Met." The cover letter indicates that unless the noncompliant CoPs are corrected within 23 calendar days, the hospital's Medicare status will be terminated. The administrator calls an emergency meeting of all affected department and service heads, and asks you to present a plan for responding to the Statement of Deficiencies. It is clear he thinks that submitting a corrective action plan will stop the termination process.

What are the elements of your presentation?

Next steps

This case is an example of what typically can happen when negative issues become survey issues. There are too many unique factors that are not mentioned here for the sake of brevity. But you know that any negative outcomes should cause you and your facility's QAPI program to start asking a lot of questions. If it doesn't, get some help to find out why. Let's talk about how CMS has decided in the fictitious case to assess the CoPs designated, and some questions they might have asked:

Governing Body:

- How does the governing body oversee the QAPI program?

- How does it approve and oversee medical staff bylaws rules and regulations?

- How does it oversee the hospital departments and services?

- How does it monitor and ensure compliance with Patients' Rights?

- Was this death in restraints reported on a timely basis to CMS?

Medical Staff:

- What role did physician management play in the case?

- Were physical restraints needed or appropriate?

- Does the medical staff have policies or rules for restraint orders that are compliant with CMS requirements (note especially the physician assessment requirements of the restraint standard)?

- Were physician orders for restraint in accordance with CMS requirements?

- Was the planned physician assessment timely and in accordance with medical staff bylaws?

- Do the bylaws address the issues in this case?

Nursing Services:

- Did staff in both the ED and on the floor follow appropriate nursing policies for restraint application, management, and assessment?

- Were assessments routinely performed accordingly to policy and on a timely basis?

- What level of monitoring was need for this patient, and was it implemented?

- Do policies address all of these issues?

Emergency Services:

- Was treatment appropriate and given by trained staff?

- Was treatment initiated promptly for this unstable patient?

- Were policies on restraint followed, and did staff follow guidelines for the decision to apply restraints in the first place?

Patients' Rights: This is pretty obvious, but certainly the restraint standard is paramount here. However, don't forget some important points in this CoP. Let's cover a few that could come up:

- Were there any indicators for pain management?

- Although the patient might have been considered incompetent to participate in any decision making in this regard, how does your hospital handle this issue?

- Might the pharmacological management of the patient's pain and behavior been a better alternative in this case? The chart and a good clinical review can hopefully tell you this.

- Was the grievance policy followed?

- Although the administrator might have thought he smoothed things over, did he follow policy?

- Is there a summary of what he said to the family, and were there witnesses? Did he consult house counsel before speaking to the family? Sometimes after relatives talk to lawyers, they change their mind about accepting apologies.

- What are the standards for protecting and enhancing patient safety?

- Even if there is an existing restraint policy, did it benefit the patient in this case?

QAPI:

- Does the QAPI program routinely gather data on restraints and patient care outcomes?

- Did it show any precursors to this case that could be linked to a failure in the system to identify the problems?

- Were QAPI activities of such a scope and nature as to be reviewing the issues found in this case?

- How is corrective action developed, implemented, and monitored by the QAPI process?

If it isn't apparent that this survey make take a while, consume a lot of hospital resources in terms of staff time, and is a very serious matter, then you need to really reconsider what you are facing. First off, you probably are at Condition-level noncompliance before the surveyors cross the threshold. You ask, "Isn't that violating our rights to have a full review before a conclusion is drawn?" Yes, but the fact that the patient has died in restraints puts you behind the proverbial eight ball from the start. Remember that patients are not supposed to die in restraints. Sound far-fetched? Your colleagues in skilled nursing facilities would tell you no one should have a decubitus ulcer in their facility according to the CMS surveyors. Your hospital is no different when it comes to this issue. Although there may be mitigating circumstances, you still should prepare for the worst in this situation, but hope for the best.

What Really Needs to be Presented (and Done)

Much of the response to an adverse event such as the one described in this case study is directly related to how well you are prepared. Regardless of the type of survey being conducted, you should have some reasonable inkling of when CMS might show up. In this case, let's cover some immediate responses that should have occurred immediately after the event, and before CMS darkens your door:

1. Mobilization of any of the affected departments and services. Forming a special ad hoc committee to develop action plans to investigate the case, propose recommendations for any changes, and pull together any evidentiary information (including interviews). Key to this process is the designation of specific personnel in each department or service who will be able to address questions from the CMS surveyors and provide them with what they need, and be able to clarify hospital policies and procedures for their area.

2. Immediate corrective action should be developed and submitted to the QAPI Committee (or the committee responsible for this function) as soon as possible. Staff of the affected departments and services should be in the process of developing written corrective action through the QAPI process.

3. Remember that corrective action may not mitigate a determination of non compliance with the COPs but it can be submitted AND implemented much more quickly if it has been developed through the QAI process immediately after the event.

4. Don't hesitate to be negative. You should act under the same assumption as CMS: The patient should not have died in restraints. Then work to prove that what was done met standards and there is no other possible explanation or action that could have been taken or given for the

mortality. It is probable, however, that your good QAPI program will find some things that need fixing. Due to the litigious nature of our society, hospitals often spend much time on defensive actions following an adverse event of this nature, and fail to recognize the opportunities that even a negative event like this can offer.

5. A plan of correction does not a correction make. Simply put, you must implement and monitor corrective action that fixes all the deficiencies identified by CMS in the CoPs that are out of compliance. You must provide corrective action for all deficiencies found on the Statement of Deficiencies. While in this case you may need to concentrate on the noncompliant CoPs, don't forget to develop and implement effective corrective action for every deficiency found. If you don't, those can develop into bigger problems later on, and the surveyors will check your surveillance history to see if there are patterns of noncompliance. Then you have a CoP out of compliance that you should have seen coming.

6. Time is not on your side. Although you may have an exit conference with the surveyors, they most often will not tell you about any potential CoP noncompliance. This can lead to false expectations and complacency. Surveyors are told not to indicate Condition-level noncompliance at the exit unless they hand you a Statement of Deficiencies at the close of the survey. Unless they are technologically astute, and the main office has approved handing out a Statement of Deficiencies that quickly, you won't know until days or even weeks after the survey.

7. As part of the overall QAPI response, include review of any corrective action plan by the QAPI process before it is submitted to CMS. This must be an integrated effort of many people who not only must provide correction action input, but also must implement the corrective action being proposed. Also remember that CMS may not accept your corrective action, so it is important to keep in touch with the surveyors as you develop the corrective action. If they don't want to talk to you (which should be an unusual situation) make sure you document your requests for your review of any draft or proposed corrective action.

8. Make corrective action permanent. Expect big trouble if you don't.

This case study was meant to show what can happen to an accredited or nonaccredited hospital when an adverse event occurs, or in general, when CMS or its state agencies conduct an allegation survey. These surveys are often built on an individual case or problem, but will be extended into compliance for each CoP chosen to be surveyed.

CMS Surveyor Guidelines for Determining Immediate Jeopardy

CMS Surveyor Guidelines for Determining Immediate Jeopardy

Editor's note: The following is excerpted from "Appendix Q: Determining Immediate Jeopardy" *of the CMS' State Operations Manual for surveyors.*

Preamble

Changes made to *Guidelines for Determining Immediate Jeopardy* reflect CMS' concern that crisis situations in which the health and safety of individuals are at risk, are accurately identified, thoroughly investigated, and resolved as quickly as possible. In the interest of consistency, the new guidelines standardize the definitions of immediate jeopardy, abuse and neglect across all certified Medicare/Medicaid entities (excluding CLIA), and describe the process surveyors use in making a determination of immediate jeopardy. The guidelines provide a detailed analysis of the steps surveyors should follow to assist them in accurately identifying those circumstances that constitute immediate jeopardy: preparation, investigation, decision-making and implementation. "Triggers" alert surveyors that some circumstances may have the potential to be identified as immediate jeopardy situations and therefore require further investigation before any determination is made. A detailed review of three sample cases walk surveyors through the steps necessary to carefully analyze and accurately determine whether or not an immediate jeopardy situation exists. To provide further guidance to surveyors, Attachment B uses actual examples of situations in which immediate jeopardy has been cited.

In the interest of reducing or eliminating abuse and neglect to all beneficiaries, the guidelines caution surveyors that when abuse or neglect has been identified, the circumstances must be thoroughly evaluated to determine if immediate jeopardy exists.

The guidelines also clarify that actual harm, as well as the potential for harm, to one or to more than one individual may constitute immediate jeopardy.

Introduction

Immediate jeopardy is interpreted as a crisis situation in which the health and safety of individual(s) are at risk. These guidelines are for use in determining if circumstances pose an immediate jeopardy to an individual's health and safety. These guidelines will assist federal and state survey and certification personnel and complaint investigators in recognizing situations that may cause or permit immediate jeopardy.

These guidelines apply to all certified Medicare/Medicaid entities (excluding the Clinical Laboratory Improvement Amendments program) and to all types of surveys and investigations: certifications, recertifications, revisits, and complaint investigations. In these guidelines, "entity" applies to all Medicare/Medicaid certified providers, suppliers, and facilities. "Surveyor" represents both surveyors and complaint investigators. "Team" represents either a single surveyor or multiple surveyors. The term "immediate jeopardy" replaces the terms "immediate and serious threat" and "serious and immediate threat" for all certified Medicare/Medicaid entities.

Note: The primary goals of these immediate jeopardy guidelines are to identify and to prevent serious injury, harm, impairment, or death.

Definitions

The following definitions apply to all certified Medicare/Medicaid entities:

Immediate jeopardy—A situation in which the provider's noncompliance with one or more requirements of participation has caused, or is likely to cause, serious injury, harm, impairment, or death to a resident.

Abuse—The willful infliction of injury, unreasonable confinement, intimidation, or punishment with resulting physical harm, pain, or mental anguish.

Neglect—Failure to provide goods and services necessary to avoid physical harm, mental anguish, or mental illness.

Principles

The goal of the survey process is to ensure the provision of quality care to all individuals receiving care or services from a certified Medicare/Medicaid entity. The identification and removal of immediate jeopardy, either psychological or physical, are essential to prevent serious harm, injury, impairment, or death for individuals.

Principles to follow include:

- Only one individual needs to be at risk. Identification of immediate jeopardy for one individual will prevent risk to other individuals in similar situations.

- Serious harm, injury, impairment, or death does not have to occur before considering immediate jeopardy. The high potential for these outcomes to occur in the very near future also constitutes immediate jeopardy.

- Individuals must not be subjected to abuse by anyone including, but not limited to, entity staff, consultants or volunteers, family members, or visitors.

- Serious harm can result from both abuse and neglect.

- Psychological harm is as serious as physical harm.

- When a surveyor has established through investigation that a cognitively impaired individual harmed an individual receiving care and services from the entity due to the entity's failure to provide care and services to avoid physical harm, mental anguish, or mental illness, this should be considered neglect.

- Any time a team cites abuse or neglect, it should consider immediate jeopardy.

Upon recognizing a situation that may constitute immediate jeopardy, the investigation process must proceed until it confirms or rules out immediate jeopardy. The serious harm, injury, impairment, or death may have occurred in the past, may be occurring at present, or may be likely to occur in the very near future as a result of the jeopardy situation. After determining that the harm meets the definition of immediate jeopardy, consider the following points regarding entity compliance:

- The entity either created a situation or allowed a situation to continue which resulted in serious harm or a potential for serious harm, injury, impairment or death to individuals.

- The entity had an opportunity to implement corrective or preventive measures.

After recognizing immediate jeopardy and completing the investigation, the team will then choose the specific federal regulation(s) to address the deficient practice. Although a specific federal regulation may not be found for each situation, all Medicare/Medicaid entities have a responsibility to provide quality care. The principles of immediate jeopardy apply to all certified entities and need to be followed for all individuals receiving care and services in those entities. The team should determine which federal regulation(s) are relevant in documenting the deficient practices(s).

Note: The key factor in the use of immediate jeopardy termination authority is, as the name implies, limited to immediate jeopardy. Immediate jeopardy procedures must not be used to enforce compliance quickly on more routine deficiencies.

Immediate jeopardy triggers

This guide lists issues with associated triggers. The issues include general statements of practices such as "Failure to protect from abuse." The guide includes situations that most likely create jeopardy to an individual's psychological/physical health and safety.

Triggers that will assist the surveyor in considering immediate jeopardy accompany each issue. Triggers describe situations that will cause the surveyor to consider if further investigation is needed to determine the presence of immediate jeopardy. The listed triggers do not automatically equal immediate jeopardy. The team must investigate and use professional judgment to determine if the situation has caused or is likely to cause serious harm, injury, impairment or death. These triggers are general examples and are not all-inclusive. Many triggers may apply to more than one issue. A trigger for an issue such as C, "Failure to Protect from Psychological Harm," could well be an example of A, "Failure to Prevent Abuse," or B, "Failure to Prevent Neglect." The team must rely on professional judgment and utilize the resources of the state survey agency, the regional CMS office, and, in the case of Medicaid-only facilities, the state Medicaid agency to determine the presence of immediate jeopardy.

Note: Harm does not have to occur before considering immediate jeopardy. Consider both potential and actual harm when reviewing the triggers in the table.

Triggers

Issue	Triggers
A. Failure to protect from abuse	1. Serious injuries such as head trauma or fractures 2. Non consensual sexual interactions (e.g., sexual harassment, sexual coercion, or sexual assault) 3. Unexplained serious injuries that have not been investigated 4. Staff striking or roughly handling an individual 5. Staff yelling, swearing, gesturing, or calling an individual derogatory names 6. Bruises around the breast or genital area or suspicious injuries (e.g., black eyes, rope marks, cigarette burns, unexplained bruising)

Triggers

Issue	Triggers
B. Failure to prevent neglect	1. Lack of timely assessment of individuals after injury
	2. Lack of supervision for individual with known special needs
	3. Failure to carry out doctor's orders
	4. Repeated occurrences such as falls which place the individual at risk of harm without intervention
	5. Access to chemical and physical hazards by individuals who are at risk
	6. Access to hot water of sufficient temperature to cause tissue injury
	7. Nonfunctioning call system without compensatory measures
	8. Unsupervised smoking by an individual with a known safety risk
	9. Lack of supervision of cognitively impaired individuals with known elopement risk
	10. Failure to adequately monitor individuals with known severe self-injurious behavior
	11. Failure to adequately monitor and intervene for serious medical/surgical conditions
	12. Use of chemical/physical restraints without adequate monitoring
	13. Lack of security to prevent abduction of infants
	14. Improper feeding/positioning of individual with known aspiration risk
	15. Inadequate supervision to prevent physical altercations

Triggers

Issue	Triggers
C. Failure to protect from psychological harm	1. Application of chemical/physical restraints without clinical indications 2. Presence of behaviors by staff such as threatening or demeaning, resulting in displays of fear, unwillingness to communicate, and recent or sudden changes in behavior by individuals 3. Lack of intervention to prevent individuals from creating an environment of fear
D. Failure to protect from undue adverse medication consequences/ failure to provide medications as prescribed	1. Administration of medication to an individual with a known history of allergic reaction to that medication 2. Lack of monitoring and identification of potential serious drug interaction, side effects, and adverse reactions 3. Administration of contraindicated medications 4. Pattern of repeated medication errors without intervention 5. Lack of diabetic monitoring resulting or likely to result in serious hypoglycemic or hyperglycemic reaction 6. Lack of timely and appropriate monitoring required for drug titration

Triggers	
Issue	**Triggers**
E. Failure to provide adequate nutrition and hydration to support and maintain health	1. Food supply inadequate to meet the nutritional needs of the individual 2. Failure to provide adequate nutrition and hydration resulting in malnutrition (e.g., severe weight loss, abnormal laboratory values) 3. Withholding nutrition and hydration without advance directive 4. Lack of potable water supply
F. Failure to protect from widespread nosocomial infections (e.g., failure to practice standard precautions, failure to maintain sterile techniques during invasive procedures, and/or failure to identify and treat nosocomial infections)	1. Pervasive improper handling of body fluids or substances from an individual with an infectious disease 2. High number of infections or contagious diseases without appropriate reporting, intervention and care 3. Pattern of ineffective infection control precautions 4. High number of nosocomial infections caused by cross contamination from staff and/or equipment/supplies

Triggers

Issue	Triggers
G. Failure to correctly identify individuals.	1. Blood products given to wrong individual 2. Surgical procedure/treatment performed on wrong individual or wrong body part 3. Administration of medication or treatments to wrong individual 4. Discharge of an infant to the wrong individual
H. Failure to safely administer blood products and safely monitor organ transplantation	1. Wrong blood type transfused 2. Improper storage of blood products 3. High number of serious blood reactions 4. Incorrect cross match and utilization of blood products or transplantation organs 5. Lack of monitoring for reactions during transfusions

Triggers	
Issue	**Triggers**
I. Failure to provide safety from fire, smoke and environment hazards, and/or failure to educate staff in handling emergency situations	1. Nonfunctioning or lack of emergency equipment/power source 2. Smoking in high risk areas 3. Incidents such as electrical shock, fires 4. Ungrounded/unsafe electrical equipment 5. Widespread lack of knowledge of emergency procedures by staff 6. Widespread infestation by insects/rodents 7. Lack of functioning ventilation, heating or cooling system placing individuals at risk 8. Use of nonapproved space heaters, such as kerosene, electrical, in resident or patient areas 9. Improper handling/disposal of hazardous materials, chemicals and waste 10. Locking exit doors in a manner that does not comply with NFPA 101 11. Obstructed hallways and exits preventing egress 12. Lack of maintenance of fire or life safety systems 13. Unsafe dietary practices resulting in high potential for foodborne illnesses

Triggers	
Issue	**Triggers**
J. Failure to provide initial medical screening, stabilization of emergency medical conditions and safe transfer for individuals and women in active labor seeking emergency treatment (Emergency Medical Treatment and Active Labor Act)	1. Individuals turned away from ER without medical screening exam 2. Women with contractions not medically screened for status of labor 3. Absence of ER and OB medical screening records 4. Failure to stabilize emergency medical condition 5. Failure to appropriately transfer an individual with an unstabilized emergency medical condition

Procedures

Preparation

The team should be familiar with these guidelines. The guidelines should be foremost in the team's mind to decrease the potential for missing immediate jeopardy. The team should also be familiar with the recommended key components of an entity's systemic approach to prevent abuse and neglect. The seven key components include: screening, training, prevention, identification, investigation, protection, and reporting/response. Both the guidelines and the key components apply to all certified Medicare/Medicaid entities.

Investigation

The investigation must be conducted in an impartial, objective manner to obtain accurate data sufficient to support a reasonable conclusion.

As you conduct the investigation, keep the following in mind:

1. Observation is a key component of any investigation. All observations need to be thoroughly documented. Be specific in noting time, location, and exact observations.

2. The interview notes must be clear and detailed. The documentation should include the full name of the person interviewed. The time and date of the interview should be documented. Any witnesses present should be indicated.

3. Record review is used to support observations and interviews. Obtain copies of relevant documentation supporting the immediate jeopardy as you investigate (e.g., nurses' notes, and investigation reports).

4. If the case involves a potential criminal action, the surveyor should be aware that any physical evidence must be preserved for law enforcement agencies.

5. Team actions:

    a. Notify the team leader immediately when an immediate jeopardy situation is suspected. The team leader will then coordinate the investigative efforts.

    b. Contact the state survey agency.

    c. Gather information to address who, what, when, where, and why. When answering these questions, consider the following:

    Who: Who was involved in the immediate jeopardy situation: staff, individuals receiving care and services, and others? Does the individual(s) at risk have special needs? Has this happened to other individuals? If yes, how many? Are there others to whom this is likely to occur? If so, how many and who? Which entity staff knew or should have known about the situation?

What: What harm has occurred, is occurring, or most likely will occur? How serious is the potential/actual harm? How did the situation occur? What was the sequence of events? What attempts did the entity make to assess, plan, correct, and reevaluate regarding the potential/actual harm? What did the entity do to prevent any further occurrences of the same nature?

When: When did the situation first occur? How long has the situation existed? Has a similar occurrence happened before? Has the entity had an opportunity to correct the situation? Did the entity thoroughly investigate the event? Did you agree with the facility's conclusion after their investigation? Did the entity implement corrective measures to prevent any further similar situations? Did they follow up and evaluate the effectiveness of their measures?

Where: Where did the potential/actual harm occur? Is this an isolated incident or an entity-wide problem?

Why: Why did the potential/actual harm occur? Was the immediate jeopardy preventable? Is there a system in place to prevent further occurrences? Is this a repeat deficient practice? Is there a pattern of similar deficient practices?

The team then needs to proceed to validate the gathered information with facility staff.

Following are two examples of teams gathering information during the investigation to answer the questions: who, what, when, where and why.

Example case #1: The resident was admitted following a hospitalization for psychiatric care. The resident had a history of exiting behavior, impulsiveness, and impaired cognition and judgment. Diagnoses included dementia with psychosis and delusion, psychomotor agitation, acute behavioral disturbances, and possible right cerebral vascular accident (CVA). Documented behavior of standing by the facility door waiting for someone to open the door and then sneaking out very fast was included in the chart.

Trigger: Lack of supervision of cognitively impaired individuals with known elopement risk.

Investigation:

Who: Who is the resident? Is the resident cognitively impaired with poor decision-making skills? Is the resident's diagnosis pertinent in this case? Is the resident physically impaired? What is the resident's ambulatory status? Was the resident identified by the facility as a wanderer oblivious to physical and safety needs? Does the resident have a history of leaving the facility without informing the staff? Does the resident's care plan address wandering and risk for elopement? Does the resident wear a safety alarm device? Is there a history of elopement from this facility? How many residents were/are at risk for elopement?

What: What happened? What was the resident's physical, mental, and emotional status prior to elopement? Was the resident injured? Did the facility seek outside medical treatment for the resident? If so, what did the reports from the ER physician's exam include regarding the resident's condition when examined?

When: When was the resident last seen? When did the resident leave the facility? When did the facility take action? When was the resident found? Who found the resident? Was the potential for injury present? Was the outdoor temperature excessively hot or cold? Was it raining, snowing, or storming, etc.? If excessively cold temperatures were present, what was the wind chill factor? How was the resident dressed? What areas of the skin were exposed and for how long?

Where: Where did the resident reside? Was the resident on a special unit with extra elopement precautions? Where did this happen? How did the resident exit the facility? Describe the exact location of exit. Where is the facility located (urban or rural)? What hazards were present in the vicinity of the facility (railroad, high motor vehicle traffic, construction zones, farm fields, lakes, ponds, etc.)?

Why: Why did this happen? Was the care plan followed? Were door alarms working properly? Were exit doors visible at all times? If so, by whom? What was the facility's plan to supervise the resident? Was it followed? If so, why did it fail? What was the physician's version of the cause for harm? Were crucial medications involving therapeutic blood/serum levels involved in the elopement (i.e., insulin, psychotropic, antihypertensives, etc.)? What other contributing factors, such as diagnosis, should be considered?

Example case #2: Confused, debilitated 75-year-old female admitted as an inpatient to the hospital has orders to discontinue all nutrition and hydration support.

Trigger: Withholding nutrition and hydration without sufficient documentation of advance directives could be an immediate jeopardy situation.

Investigation:

Who: Who wrote the order? Is this the patient's primary care physician? Who has the authority to make the medical care decisions? Does the patient have a living will? Does the patient have a durable power of attorney? Who has spoken with the person designated to make healthcare decisions for the patient (e.g., social worker, primary care physician, specialist, hospice nurse, or chaplain)?

What: What is the patient's diagnosis? Is documentation of a terminal disease process by the attending physician contained in the progress notes? What does the progress note contain about risks and benefits of discontinuation of hydration and nutrition? What alternative treatment options have been considered and discussed with the person responsible for making healthcare decisions for this patient? What events precipitated the decision to discontinue hydration and nutrition? What care and services have been planned during the absence of nutrition and hydration? What steps have been taken to ascertain the patient's wishes? What is state law regarding advance directives and end-of-life issues?

When: When did the hospital obtain evidence of the patient's wishes regarding end of life treatment? When did the physician discuss end of life issues, diagnosis, prognosis and the patient's wishes with the person designated by the patient or by law to make healthcare decisions?

Where: If the patient has an advance directive, how easy/difficult is it to find in the chart to verify the patient's wishes? If the advance directive is not in the chart, does the chart indicate where the advance directive is kept? If the patient does not have an advance directive, where is the documentation in the chart to support the patient's wishes to discontinue nutrition and hydration at the end of life? Where is the documentation to support that the person making the healthcare decisions is fully informed of the risks and benefits, and is making the decisions the patient would have made? If the patient does not have an advance directive, does the patient's chart reflect compliance with the State law and the legal representative's decision-making authority concerning withdrawal of hydration and nutrition? Has the person with decision-making authority been fully informed of all options, including home care, hospice, and long-term care placement?

Why: If the physician wrote an order to discontinue nutrition and hydration, does the progress note contain documentation of the rationale? Is there clear documentation to support the decision?

The decision process

The information gathered is used to evaluate the provision of related care and services, occurrence frequency, and the likelihood of repetition. The team needs to have gathered and validated sufficient information to address the three components of immediate jeopardy to begin the decision process.

Components of immediate jeopardy

1. Harm

   a. **Actual**—Was there an outcome of harm? Does the harm meet the definition of immediate jeopardy (e.g., has the provider's noncompliance caused serious injury, harm, impairment, or death to an individual)?

   b. **Potential**—Is there a likelihood of potential harm? Does the potential harm meet the definition of immediate jeopardy (e.g., is the provider's noncompliance likely to cause serious injury, harm, impairment, or death to an individual)?

2. **Immediacy**—Is the harm or potential harm likely to occur in the very near future to this individual or others in the entity, if immediate action is not taken?

3. **Culpability**

   a. Did the entity know about the situation? If so, when did the entity first become aware?

   b. Should the entity have known about the situation?

   c. Did the entity thoroughly investigate the circumstances?

   d. Did the entity implement corrective measures?

   e. Has the entity reevaluated the measures to ensure the situation was corrected?

Note: The team must consider the entity's response to any harm or potential harm that meets the definition of immediate jeopardy. The stated lack of knowledge by the entity about a particular situation does not excuse an entity from knowing and preventing immediate jeopardy. The team should use knowledge and experience to determine if the circumstances could have been predicted. The immediate jeopardy investigation should proceed until the team has gathered enough information to evaluate any prior indications or warnings regarding the jeopardy situation and the entity's response. The crisis situations in which an entity did not have any prior indications or warnings, and could not have predicted a potential serious harm, are very rare.

Team actions

Team actions include the following:

- Meet as a team.

- Follow these guidelines.

- Share collected data.

- Identify the three components of immediate jeopardy.

- Decide if you have enough information to make a decision. If not, continue the investigation.

- Identify any inconsistencies or contradictions between interviews, observations and record reviews.

- Clarify any inconsistencies or contradictions.

- Determine the specific federal regulation for the situation.

- Consult with the state agency, as necessary.

The following are examples of decision-making as the team analyzes the information obtained during the investigation.

Example case #1 (continued): During the survey, the resident was observed to enter the code and exit the unit without assistance five times in 30 minutes and was brought back by nursing staff from the unit, nursing staff from other units and administrative staff. The front door to the facility had a broken alarm and did not latch properly and was easily accessible after exiting the locked unit. The facility was aware of the broken alarm and latch. The chart contained documentation that the facility was aware of the resident's ability to operate the door keypads for at least 60 days. The facility was located in an urban area on a busy street. A row of trees prevented anyone in the facility from viewing a resident exiting the property and crossing the street.

The record included documentation of the resident exiting the building successfully without notice. The documentation included only a brief description of the incident. After a search, the resident was located in an area emergency room being treated for a minor laceration of the lip. Police notified the facility that bystanders who had called 911 had found the resident lying down with blood on her face. The chart included subsequent reports of repeated frequent attempts to elope 25–40 times per shift, and the statement, "Patient requires 1:1, care not safe on this unit secondary to continuous exit seeking." A review of the facility investigations revealed that the facility had not completed any investigations for this resident.

Decision-making:

Consider the following during the decision-making process:

- Has actual harm occurred? Yes.

- Does the actual harm that occurred meet the definition of immediate jeopardy? No.

- Is there a likelihood of potential serious harm? Yes.

- Does the potential harm meet the definition of immediate jeopardy? Yes.

- Is the harm likely to recur in the very near future, if immediate action is not taken? Yes.

- Did the facility have knowledge of the situation? Yes. If so, when did they first become aware? Before admission when notified of history.

- Did the facility thoroughly investigate the circumstances? No.

- Did the facility implement corrective measures? No.

- Does this meet the definition of immediate jeopardy? Yes.

- Which is the most appropriate tag to define the failed practice?

Outcome:

The investigation's outcome is as follows:

- The team identifies the most appropriate regulation that applies to the situation.

- The team proceeds with documentation of the immediate jeopardy deficient practice.

- The state agency proceeds with the termination procedures per the CMS' *State Operations Manual*.

- Except in the case of Medicaid-only facilities, the CMS regional office proceeds with termination actions.

Example case #2 (continued): During the investigation, the surveyor finds that the chart does not include a copy of the patient's advance directive. The progress note does not contain any documentation of the patient ever stating a wish to have nutrition and hydration withdrawn at the end of life. The patient has a diagnosis of advance dementia with a documented history of refusal to eat in a long-term care facility. The patient had been admitted because of continued weight loss and dehydration related to the refusal to eat or drink. The patient has a daughter who actively participates in her mother's care, is identified as the legal representative, and is identified in the social service notes as the closest living family member. The primary care physician documented a discussion with the daughter concerning the patient's poor prognosis for meaningful recovery. Although death is not imminent as a result of the dementia, death is the expected result at some unknown time in the future. The chart does not include any documentation that the daughter expressed a wish to have nutrition and hydration support withdrawn. The social worker was unable to confirm that the daughter had expressed a wish to have all support withdrawn. The social worker is uncertain why the nutrition and hydration were discontinued. When contacted, the daughter is unaware that support has been withdrawn and is very upset. The surveyor copies the order sheet, the progress notes and the social service notes. The surveyor clearly documents the interviews with the social worker and the daughter. There is a discrepancy between the written order for withdrawal of support and the daughter's and the social worker's knowledge of the situation. The surveyor decides to present the information to the team prior to contacting the physician.

Decision-making:

Consider the following during the decision-making process:

- Has actual harm occurred? No.

- Is there a likelihood of potential serious harm? Yes.

- Does the potential serious harm meet the definition of immediate jeopardy (e.g., serious injury, harm, impairment, or death)? Yes.

- Is the potential serious harm likely to occur in the very near future, if immediate action is not taken? Yes.

- Did the facility have knowledge of the situation? Yes.

If so, when did the facility first become aware? After the doctor's order was written?

- Did the facility thoroughly investigate the circumstances? No.

- Did the facility implement corrective measures? No.

- Does this meet the definition of immediate jeopardy? Yes.

- Which is the most appropriate tag to define the failed practice?

Outcome:

The investigation's outcome is as follows:

- The team identifies the most appropriate regulation that applies to the situation.

- The team proceeds with documentation of the immediate jeopardy deficient practice.

- The state agency proceeds with the termination procedures per the *CMS' State Operations Manual*.

- The CMS regional office proceeds with termination actions.

Example case #3: An outside intruder entered a resident's room by cutting through the screen. A resident with a diagnosis of advanced dementia was raped. The resident did not notify staff at the time of the incident. The intruder was not observed entering the facility by any facility staff. However, nightshift staff immediately called the police after noticing a stranger in the courtyard at the back of the facility. The police came and were unable to locate anyone. The police checked the grounds without incident and then encouraged the staff to check the locks on the doors and windows and obtain services to monitor the premises for increased security. The police indicated that no prior intruders had been reported in the neighborhood.

The facility immediately contacted a local security service and hired a security guard to monitor the outside grounds. The security guard arrived within 45 minutes and began patrolling the grounds. The facility staff checked all the doors and windows to ensure security. They checked on all of the residents and did not observe any problems. During morning rounds, the resident reported that someone had hurt her during the night. The staff noted that the screen had been damaged and immediately contacted the police and the state agency. The police came and had the resident transported to the nearest emergency room for a rape assessment. The emergency room confirmed that the resident had been raped.

Decision-making:

Consider the following during the decision-making process:

- Has actual harm occurred? Yes.

- Does the harm meet the definition of immediate jeopardy (e.g., serious injury, harm, impairment, or death to an individual)? Yes.

- Is the harm likely to recur in the very near future, if immediate action is not taken? Yes.

- Did the entity have knowledge of the situation? Yes.

If so, when did the entity first become aware? In the morning when the resident reported she had been hurt.

- Did the entity thoroughly investigate the circumstances? Yes.

- Did they implement corrective measures? Yes.

- Does this meet the definition of immediate jeopardy? No. The facility reacted appropriately and followed the recommendations of the law enforcement experts to protect all residents. The harm to the resident had already occurred before the facility had any indications or warnings, and could not have been predicted or prevented.

Outcome:

The investigation's outcome is as follows:

- The team gathered sufficient data to reach the conclusion that the facility had no predictable way of knowing that residents were at risk for harm from an intruder.

- The team also gathered sufficient data to reach a decision that the facility reacted immediately to protect residents when they had knowledge of a potential risk.

- The team concludes that there was no failed practice.

- The team concludes its investigation of this complaint.

Implementation

Team actions

If the team reaches a consensus concerning the presence of immediate jeopardy, the team leader then contacts the state agency per the protocol established by the state agency. Expedite the state agency review. If the team is unable to follow the state agency protocol for administrative consultation, actions to proceed with implementation of immediate jeopardy must continue. Decide if any other agencies need to be notified (e.g., law enforcement agency, nurses' aide registration board).

Note: Any criminal act must be reported to the local law enforcement agency. The entity should be encouraged to make the report, if needed. The surveyor should only assume this responsibility if the entity refuses.

State agency actions

Upon review of the findings, if the state agency concurs with the team's consensus of immediate jeopardy, the state agency will inform the CMS regional office for all Medicare and dually certified entities. For Medicaid-only facilities, the state agency will notify the state Medicaid agency. For immediate jeopardy in Medicaid-only facilities, contact the regional office per the protocol established between the state agency and the regional office.

Team action

Once the team has decided that immediate jeopardy exists, the team should notify the administration of the immediate jeopardy. A verbal notice should be given with the specific details, including the individuals at risk, before the survey team leaves the premises of the entity. The entity should begin immediate removal of the risk to individuals, and immediately implement corrective measures to prevent repeat jeopardy situations. The team should encourage the entity to provide evidence of their implementation of corrective measures.

The notice describing the immediate jeopardy must be delivered to the entity no later than two days from the end of the survey. If official notification of all deficiencies (i.e., form CMS-2567) was not given on the second day, a completed form CMS-2567 must be sent to the entity on the 10th working day.

Documentation

Skilled nursing facilities/nursing facilities (SNF/NF)

Consider the following documentation guidelines:

1—Confirmation of removal of immediate jeopardy

Only on-site confirmation of implementation of the facility's corrective actions justifies a determination that the immediate jeopardy has been removed.

2—Immediate jeopardy removed, deficient practice corrected

If the facility is able to remove the immediate jeopardy before the survey team leaves the facility and to correct associated deficient practices, cite the immediate jeopardy at the immediate jeopardy severity and scope (J, K, or L). Document evidence of the facility's actions, including dates that indicate that the facility has removed the immediate jeopardy and corrected the deficient practice. The date of full correction will be shown on the Form CMS-2567B.

3—Immediate jeopardy removed, deficient practice present

If the facility is able to employ immediate corrective measures that remove the immediate jeopardy, but an associated deficient practice still exists at a lesser severity and scope, cite the immediate jeopardy at the immediate jeopardy severity and scope. Include the documentation to support the remaining deficient practice. Document the level of harm and the identified residents in the Statement of Deficiencies. Attach the corrective measures submitted by the facility as an immediate plan of correction.

4—Immediate jeopardy not removed

If the facility is unable or unwilling to remove the immediate jeopardy before the end of the survey, inform the administration that the CMS regional office will be notified of the immediate jeopardy and termination procedures will be initiated. Use the appropriate *State Operations Manual* reference to define the end of the survey.

All entities not noted above

Immediate jeopardy is always cited at the Condition level on the Form CMS-2567.

1—Confirmation of removal of immediate jeopardy

Only on-site confirmation of implementation of the facility's corrective action justifies a determination that the immediate jeopardy has been removed.

2 - Immediate jeopardy removed, deficient practice corrected

If the entity is able to remove the immediate jeopardy and correct associated deficient practices before the team exits, cite the immediate jeopardy at the Condition level on the Form CMS-2567. Corrective actions taken by the provider/supplier will be included in the Form CMS-2567 documentation. The date of full correction will be shown on the Form CMS-2567B.

3—Immediate jeopardy removed, deficient practice present at Condition level

If the entity is able to employ immediate corrective measures that remove the immediate jeopardy, but an associated deficient practice still remains at the Condition level for the same Condition of Participation, cite the Condition of Participation as not met and proceed with 90-day termination procedures. Include documentation of both the immediate jeopardy with subsequent removal, and the remaining deficient practice in this citation.

4—Immediate jeopardy removed, deficient practice present at standard or elemental level

If the entity is able to employ immediate corrective measures, which remove the immediate jeopardy but an associated deficient practice still remains at the standard or elemental level, cite the immediate jeopardy at the Condition of Participation level on Form CMS-2567. Cite the remaining deficiency at the most appropriate standard or elemental tag. The date of removal of the immediate jeopardy will be shown on the Form CMS-2567B.

5—Immediate jeopardy not removed

If the entity is unable or unwilling to remove the immediate jeopardy before the team's exit, inform the administration that the CMS regional office will be notified of the immediate jeopardy situation and termination procedures will be initiated. In the case of a Medicaid-only facility, the state Medicaid agency will be notified of the immediate jeopardy.

Enforcement

A—Termination for Title XIX-only nursing facilities, intermediate care facilities for people with mental retardation

Refer to State Operations Manual §3005 E for specific instructions.

B—Enforcement for SNF/NF

Refer to State Operations Manual §§7307-7309 for specific instructions.

C—Termination for all other Medicare Entities

Refer to State Operations Manual §3010.

CMS Ambulatory Surgical Services Interpretive Guidelines

CMS Ambulatory Surgical Services Interpretive Guidelines

Editor's note: The following is excerpted from Appendix L—Guidance to Surveyors: Ambulatory Surgical Services, which is part of the CMS State Operations Manual. *The guidelines were revised May 21, 2004.*

§416.2 Definitions

Ambulatory surgical center (ASC) means any distinct entity that operates exclusively for the purpose of providing surgical services to patients not requiring hospitalization, has an agreement with CMS under Medicare to participate as an ASC, and meets the conditions set forth in Subpart B and C of this part.

Interpretive Guidelines §416.2

The ASC must use its space for ambulatory surgery exclusively. Recordkeeping must be exclusive to the ASC, and the staff must be responsible to the ASC. For example, a nurse could not provide coverage in the ASC and in an adjacent clinic (or hospital) at the same time. The ASC is not required to be in a building separate from other healthcare activities (e.g., hospital, clinic, physician's office). It must be separated physically by at least semipermanent walls and doors.

The regulatory definition of an ASC does not allow the ASC and another entity to mix functions and operations in a common space during concurrent or overlapping hours of operation. Another entity may share common space only if the space is never used during the scheduled hours of ASC operation. However, the operating and recovery rooms must be used exclusively for surgical procedures.

The ASC may not perform a surgical procedure on a Medicare patient when, before surgery, an overnight hospital stay is anticipated. There may, however, arise unanticipated medical circumstances that warrant a Medicare patient's hospitalization after an ASC surgical procedure. The ASC must have procedures for the immediate transfer of these patients to a hospital. Such situations should be infrequent.

ASC-covered procedures are those that generally do not exceed 90 minutes in length and do not require more than four hours recovery or convalescent time. Thus, ASC patients generally do not require extended care as a result of ASC procedures. An unanticipated medical circumstance may arise that would require an ASC patient to stay in an overnight healthcare setting. Such situations should be infrequent. When extended care in a nonhospital healthcare setting is anticipated as a result of a particular procedure, that procedure would not be a covered ASC procedure for Medicare beneficiaries.

§416.40 Condition for Coverage: Compliance With Licensure Law

The ASC must comply with state licensure requirements.

Interpretive Guidelines §416.40

In states where licensure is required for a facility providing ambulatory surgical services, ask to see the facility's current license. If the state license is revoked, the ASC is out of compliance with this condition. This may result in its termination from participation in Medicare. Where a state has no applicable licensure requirements, or where ambulatory surgical services may be provided without licensure, a facility will be eligible if it meets the definition in §416.2 and all other applicable Medicare requirements. Failure of the facility to meet state licensure law may be cited when the authority having jurisdiction (AHJ) has made a determination of noncompliance and has also taken a final adverse action as a result. If the surveyor identifies a situation that indicates the provider may not be in compliance with state licensure law, the information may be referred to the AHJ for follow-up. If the facility is not in compliance with state licensure law, the facility could be found out of compliance with §416.40.

Q-0003 §416.41 Condition for Coverage: Governing Body and Management

The ASC must have a governing body that assumes full legal responsibility for determining, implementing, and monitoring policies governing the ASC's total operation and for ensuring that these policies are administered so as to provide quality healthcare in a safe environment. When services are provided through a contract with an outside resource, the ASC must assure that these services are provided in a safe and effective manner.

Interpretive Guidelines §416.41

The ASC must have a designated governing body that demonstrates its oversight of ASC activities intended to protect the health and safety of patients. Consider the following:

- An individual may act as the governing body in the case of sole-ownership, absentee ownership, or in other special cases.

- Responsibilities may be formally delegated to administrative, medical, or other personnel for carrying out various activities. However, the governing body must retain ultimate responsibility.

The ASC must establish and carry out activities that will ensure that contracted services are provided in a safe manner.

Survey Procedures and Probes §416.41

Review chapter or titles of incorporation, bylaws, and partnership agreements. Annotate on the survey report form if full legal responsibilities have been established.

Q-0004 §416.41 Standard: Hospitalization

The ASC must have an effective procedure for the immediate transfer to a hospital, of patients requiring emergency medical care beyond the capabilities of the ASC. This hospital must be a local, Medicare-participating hospital or a local, nonparticipating hospital that meets the requirements for payment under §482.2 of this chapter. The ASC must have a written transfer agreement with such a hospital, or all physicians performing surgery in the ASC must have admitting privileges at such a hospital.

Interpretive Guidelines §416.41

An "effective procedure" encompasses:

- Written guidelines (e.g., policies and/or procedures)

- Arrangement for ambulance services

- Transfer of medical information

Survey Procedures and Probes §416.41

Request documentation of a transfer agreement or evidence of admitting privileges, and keep in mind the following:

- Policies and procedures must be established for transferring patients requiring emergency care.

- Appropriate personnel should be aware of transfer procedures.

Q-0005 §416.42 Condition for Coverage: Surgical Services

Surgical procedures must be performed in a safe manner by qualified physicians who have been granted clinical privileges by the governing body of the ASC in accordance with approved policies and procedures of the ASC.

Interpretive Guidelines §416.42

"In a safe manner" means that:

- The equipment and supplies are sufficient so that the type of surgery conducted can be performed in a manner that will not endanger the health and safety of the patient

- Access to operative and recovery areas is limited

- All individuals in the surgical area are to conform to aseptic techniques

- Appropriate cleaning is completed between surgical cases

- Suitable equipment is available for rapid and routine sterilization of operating room materials

- Sterilized materials are packaged, labeled, and stored in a manner to ensure sterility and that each item is marked with the expiration date

- Operating room attire is suitable for the kind of surgical cases performed

- (Persons working in the operating suite must wear clean surgical costumes in lieu of their ordinary clothing. Surgical costumes are to be designed for maximum skin and hair coverage.)

Survey Procedures and Probes §416.42

Policies and procedures should contain at a minimum:

- Resuscitative techniques

- Aseptic technique and scrub procedures

- Care of surgical specimens

- Appropriate protocols for all surgical procedures, specific or general in nature, and include a list of equipment, materials, and supplies necessary to properly

- Carry out job assignments

- Procedures addressing the cleaning of operating room after each use

- Sterilization and disinfection procedures

- Acceptable operating room attire

- Care of anesthesia equipment

- Special provision for infected or contaminated patients

Q-0006 §416.42(a) Standard: Anesthetic Risk and Evaluation

A physician must examine the patient immediately before surgery to evaluate the risk of anesthesia and of the procedure to be performed. Before discharge from the ASC, each patient must be evaluated by a physician for proper anesthesia recovery.

Survey Procedures and Probes §416.42(a)

The medical record should confirm:

- If laboratory studies were ordered as part of patient evaluation. The report should be part of the medical record or notation of the findings recorded on the chart.

- For general anesthesia, the evaluation should contain, at a minimum, a brief note regarding the heart and lung findings the day of surgery

- Depending on the type of anesthesia and length of surgery, the postoperative check should include some or all of the following:
  - Level of activity
  - Respirations
  - Blood pressure
  - Level of consciousness
  - Patient color

Q-0007 §416.42(b) Standard: Administration of Aesthesia

Anesthesia must be administered by only:

(1) A qualified anesthesiologist, or

(2) A physician qualified to administer anesthesia, a certified registered nurse anesthetist, a supervised trainee in an approved educational program, or an anesthesiologist's assistant. In those cases in which a nonphysician administers the anesthesia, the anesthetist must be under the supervision of the operating physician, and in the case of an anesthesiologist's assistant, under the supervision of an anesthesiologist.

Survey Procedures and Probes §416.42(b)

The ASC indicates those persons qualified to administer anesthesia. An approved educational program is a formal training program leading to licensure or certification in anesthesia that is recognized by the state.

Q-0008 §416.42(c) Standard: Discharge

All patients are discharged in the company of a responsible adult, except those exempted by the attending physician.

Interpretive Guidelines §416.42(c)

Any exceptions to this requirement must be made by the attending physician and annotated on the discharge plan.

Q-0009 §416.43 Condition for Coverage: Evaluation of Quality

The ASC, with the active participation of the medical staff, must conduct an ongoing, comprehensive self-assessment of the quality of care provided, including medical necessity of procedures performed and appropriateness of care, and use findings, when appropriate, in the revision of center policies and consideration of clinical privileges.

Interpretive Guidelines §416.43

Evaluation of quality of care is a rapidly evolving area. Major changes have occurred in the field of quality assurance, primarily in terminology and the methods used to monitor care. Some of the changes include:

- Increased emphasis on organizational systems and processes (rather than individual case review)

- Increased recognition of the need for objective data

- Increased use of quality indicators or performance measures with which to analyze patient care processes and outcomes

- Increased emphasis on quality monitoring for identifying opportunities to improve care (rather than focusing only on problem identification)

Indicators or performance measures are tools that monitor important clinical, management, support, and governance processes and outcomes. Ongoing monitoring of important processes and outcomes allows the ASC to measure performance in key areas and identify opportunities to improve care.

Survey Procedures and Probes §416.43

Items for discussion with facility staff may include:

- Describe an important opportunity to improve the patient care process or outcomes in the ASC.

- How did you become aware of this particular opportunity to improve patient care?

- What was done, or what would you suggest should be done, to improve the patient care process or outcome?

- Who contributed, or who would you suggest contribute, to the improvement effort?

Items for review include:

- How and when is quality monitoring conducted?

- What key indicators of quality or performance measures are monitored by the ASC?

- How does the medical staff participate in quality assurance?

- How does the ASC review appropriateness of care?

- How policies and clinical privileges are revised to improve patient care processes?

For an initial certification, there are no historical records of quality monitoring to review. However, review for evidence that the ASC has outlined a program to monitor key indicators of quality and appropriateness, and that proper reporting and accountability mechanisms are in place. For existing programs, the most important factor to evaluate is whether the ASC's quality assurance or quality improvement program has been implemented. Review the facility's program documentation and other records to determine whether patient quality of care and administrative issues that impact on quality have been identified.

The ASC should use the results of ongoing quality monitoring to identify processes that need improvement, develop and implement corrective actions and evaluate whether the problems have been eliminated or minimized. Annotate on the survey report form what the ASC considers important processes to patient care that should be evaluated ongoing, and that are not ongoing. Ongoing means that there is continuing or periodic collection and assessment of data concerning all areas that impact on patient care. The program continually identifies processes for improvement and potential problems and indicates the data that should be collected and assessed in order to provide the ASC with routine findings regarding quality of patient care.

The monitoring should be comprehensive and take into consideration medical necessity as it relates to the procedure performed by the ASC. The quality assurance or improvement program should also monitor the quality of patient education before procedures are performed and prior to discharge after the procedure. Specifically, are patients given necessary information to prepare for the procedure and to perform self-care and manage complications after discharge?

Evaluation of appropriateness of care should include analysis of:

- Anesthesia recovery

- Infection rates

- Pathology reports

- Nursing services

- Completeness of medical records

- Complications that have occurred

- Stability at discharge

There should be sufficient data in the medical records to support the diagnosis and procedures appropriate to the diagnosis. The methods use for facility self-assessment may be very flexible and there may be a wide variety of assessment techniques used. Care may be assessed prospectively, concurrently, or retrospectively. Where problems (or potential problems) are identified following the above analysis, ASCs should take appropriate action as soon as possible to avoid any risk to patients.

Examples of appropriate action may include:

- Changes in policies, processes and procedures

- Staffing and assignment changes

- Appropriate education and training

- Adjustments in clinical privileges

- Changes in equipment or physical plant

Q-0010 §416.44 Conditions for Coverage: Environment

The ASC must have a safe and sanitary environment, properly constructed, equipped, and maintained to protect the health and safety of patients.

Survey Procedures and Probes §416.44

Tour the facility and annotate on the survey report form whether the facility is adequately designed and equipped, clean and orderly, and free of hazards.

Q-0011 §416.44(a) Standard: Physical Environment

The ASC must provide a functional and sanitary environment for the provision of surgical services.

Q-0012 §416.44(a)(1)

Each operating room must be designed and equipped so that the types of surgery conducted can be performed in a manner that protects the lives and assures the physical safety of all individuals in the area.

Survey Procedures and Probes §416.44(a)

Each operating room should be designed and equipped for the types of surgery performed and free of hazards to patients and staff (e.g., sufficient space, adequate lighting, necessary furniture).

Q-0013 §416.44(a)(2)

The ASC must have a separate recovery room and waiting area.

Q-0014 §416.44(a)(3)

The ASC must establish a program for identifying and preventing infections, maintaining a sanitary environment, and reporting the results to appropriate authorities.

Interpretive Guidelines §416.44(a)(3)

Since there is a risk of nosocomial infection there must be an active surveillance program of specific measures for prevention, early detection, control, education, and investigation of infectious and communicable diseases in ASCs. There must be a mechanism to evaluate the program(s) and take corrective action.

The ASC should institute the most current recommendations of the Centers for Disease Control and Prevention (CDC) relative to the specific infection(s) and communicable disease(s).

Survey Procedures and Probes §416.44(a)(3)

Annotate on the survey report form if the written policies and procedures do not contain, at a minimum:

- Methods to minimize sources and transmission of infection, including adequate surveillance techniques such as:

  - Assessing the risk for infections and communicable diseases
  - Identifying patients at risk for infections and communicable diseases
  - Educating healthcare workers about infectious and communicable diseases
  - Screening healthcare workers
  - Providing a safe environment consistent with the most current CDC recommendations
  - Providing treatment measures consistent with the most current CDC recommendation for the identified infection/communicable disease
  - Providing for program evaluation and revision of program, when indicated

- Sterilizing techniques for supplies and equipment

- Procedures for isolation

- Procedures for orientation of all new employees in infection control and personal hygiene

- Aseptic technique procedures

Staff should have knowledge of infection control techniques and of the ASC's infection control program. The ASC should maintain an ongoing log that reports incidents of infection.

Q-0015 §416.44(b) Standard: Safety From Fire

(1) Except as provided in paragraphs (b)(2) and (3) of this section, the ASC must meet the provisions of the 1985 edition of the *Life Safety Code ® (LSC)* of the National Fire Protection Association (NFPA) that are applicable to ASCs.

(2) In consideration of a recommendation by the state survey agency, CMS may waive, for periods

deemed appropriate, specific provisions of the *LSC* which, if rigidly applied, would result in unreasonable hardship upon an ASC, but only if the waiver will not adversely affect the health and safety of the patients.

(3) Any ASC that, on May 9, 1988, complies with the requirements of the 1981 edition of the *LSC*, with or without waivers, will be considered to be in compliance with this standard, so long as the ASC continues to remain in compliance with that edition of the *LSC*.

Interpretive Guidelines §416.44(b)

The provisions of the NFPA's (1985 edition) *LSC* (unless facility is grandfathered under the 1981 *LSC* provisions prior to May 5, 1988) that apply are:

- Section 12-6 and Chapter 26, whichever provisions are more stringent, for new facilities and building permits issued or plans reviewed on or after May 5, 1988, (September 7, 1982, for facilities grandfathered under the 1981 *LSC* provisions);
  or

- Section 13-6 and Chapter 27, whichever provisions are more stringent, for facilities and building permits issued or plans reviewed prior to May 5, 1988, (September 7, 1982, for facilities grandfathered under the 1981 *LSC* provisions).

Survey Procedures and Probes §416.44(b)

The state fire authority should be used to conduct an *LSC* survey. This is usually the *LSC* unit of the state health department or the office of the state fire marshal. It is the same unit that conducts *LSC* surveys for hospitals and nursing homes.

Whenever a waiver is requested, submit documentation of "unreasonable hardship" and "no adverse effects on health safety" along with your recommendations through the state agency to the CMS regional office, which will grant or deny the waiver.

Q-0016 §416.44(c) Standard: Emergency Equipment

Emergency equipment available to the operating rooms must include at least the following:

Q-0017

§416.44(c)(1) Emergency call system

> (2) Oxygen

> (3) Mechanical ventilatory assistance, equipment including airways, manual breathing bag, and ventilator

> (4) Cardiac defibrillator

> (5) Cardiac monitoring equipment

> (6) Tracheostomy set

> (7) Laryngoscope and endotracheal tubes

> (8) Suction equipment

> (9) Emergency medical equipment and supplies specified by the medical staff

Q-0018 §416.44(d) Standard: Emergency Personnel

Personnel trained in the use of emergency equipment and in cardiopulmonary resuscitation must be available whenever there is a patient in the ASC.

Survey Procedures and Probes §416.44(d)

Request documentation of personnel trained in the use of emergency equipment and in cardiopulmonary resuscitation. Request documentation that indicates these personnel is available at all times for emergencies.

Q-0019 §416.45 Condition for Coverage: Medical Staff

The medical staff of the ASC must be accountable to the governing body.

Interpretive Guidelines §416.45

The organization of the medical staff is left to the discretion of the ASC governing body. (Membership on the governing body may include physician and nonphysician practitioners.) Privileges granted, however, must be consistent with the license to practice in the state and the experience of each clinical practitioner.

Q-0020 §416.45(a) Standard: Membership and Clinical Privileges

Members of the medical staff must be legally and professionally qualified for the positions to which they are appointed and for the performance of privileges in accordance with recommendations from qualified medical personnel.

Interpretive Guidelines §416.45(a)

The ASC is not required to follow each recommendation (e.g., acceptance or denial of privileges), but granting of privileges must be supported by recommendations.

Survey Procedures and Probes §416.45(a)

Select no more than five personnel records for medical staff members that have been granted clinical privileges and annotate on the survey report form if there is no documentation of personnel qualifications, privileges granted, appropriate records and other related documents.

Q-0021 §416.45(b) Standard: Reappraisals

Medical staff privileges must be periodically reappraised by the ASC. The scope of procedures performed in the ASC must be periodically reviewed and amended as appropriate.

Survey Procedures and Probes §416.45(b)

The policies and procedures manuals should state how often reappraisals are to be conducted.

Select no more than five personnel records for medical staff members that have been granted clinical privileges and annotate on the survey report form if there is no documentation of reappraisals being performed timely.

Q-0022 §416.45(c) Standard: Other Practitioners

If the ASC assigns patient care responsibilities to practitioners other than physicians, it must have established policies and procedures, approved by the governing body, for overseeing and evaluating their clinical activities.

Interpretive Guidelines §416.45(c)

Patient care responsibilities (which may or may not include formal privileges) may be assigned to practitioners not meeting the definition of physician in §1861(r) of the Act. However, policies and procedures must be established (e.g., either as part of overall medical staff bylaws or as separate documents) to oversee their clinical activities. "Physician" is defined in §1861(r) of the Social Security Act as:

- Doctor of medicine or osteopathy

- Doctor of dental surgery or of dental medicine

- Doctor of podiatric medicine

- Doctor of optometry with respect to services legally authorized to be performed in the state

- Chiropractor with respect to treatment by manual manipulation of the spine (to correct subluxation diagnosed by x-ray).

All of the above must practice in accordance with state licensure.

Q-0023

§416.46 Condition for Coverage: Nursing Service
The nursing services of the ASC must be directed and staffed to assure that the nursing needs of all patients are met.

Q-0024 §416.46(a) Standard: Organization and Staffing

Patient care responsibilities must be delineated for all nursing service personnel. Nursing services must be provided in accordance with recognized standards of practice. There must be a registered nurse available for emergency treatment whenever there is a patient in the ASC.

Interpretive Guidelines §416.46(a)

"Available" means on the premises and sufficiently free from other duties, enabling the individual to respond rapidly to emergency situations. Functions, qualifications, and patient care responsibilities should be delineated for all nursing personnel.

Survey Procedures and Probes §416.46(a)

Select a random sample of surgical cases. Annotate on the survey report form if registered nurses are not on-site and available for emergencies during ASC hours of operation. ASC policy must explain current acceptable standards of practice. "Recognized standards of practice" are standards promoted by national, state, and local nursing associations, relating to safe and effective nursing services.

Q-0025 §416.47 Condition for Coverage: Medical Records

The ASC must maintain complete, comprehensive, and accurate medical records to ensure adequate patient care.

Survey Procedures and Probes §416.47

Medical records should be properly indexed and readily retrievable. Make sure that medical records are protected from fire and unauthorized access, and are properly stored. The policy manual must address retention, preservation, and confidentiality of the medical records.

Q-0026 §416.47(a) Standard: Organization

The ASC must develop and maintain a system for the proper collection, storage, and use of patient records.

Survey Procedures and Probes §416.47(a)

If patient records are not collected in a systematic manner for easy access, annotate this on the survey report form. Request six patient records and observe whether the facility has a functioning medical record system that safeguards the retention of medical records.

Q-0027 §416.47(b) Standard: Form and Content of Record

The ASC must maintain a medical record for each patient. Every record must be accurate, legible, and promptly completed. Medical records must include at least the items listed below in §416.47(b).

Survey Procedures and Probes §416.47(a)

Select a random sample of records to evaluate the completeness of information, recording of treatment/services provided, and content as specified in this standard. The random sample should include a sample of records from all practitioners. If you identify specific problems or trends of incomplete records, select additional records.

Q-0028 §416.47(b)

(1) Patient identification

(2) Significant medical history and results of physical examination

(3) Preoperative diagnostic studies (entered before surgery), if performed

(4) Findings and techniques of the operation including a pathologist's report on all tissues removed during surgery, except those exempted by the governing body

(5) Any allergies and abnormal drug reactions

(6) Entries related to anesthesia administration

(7) Documentation of properly executed informed patient consent

(8) Discharge diagnosis

Survey Procedures and Probes §416.47(b)(2)

The medical history and physical examination should be relevant to the reason for surgery and the type of anesthesia planned. It should validate the need for surgery balanced against the risk factors associated with anesthesia (e.g., smoking history, problems associated with past anesthesia). Record any inconsistencies on the survey report form.

Survey Procedures and Probes §416.47(b)(4)

Request the list of approved exemptions. Exemptions to a pathology report should be made only when the quality of care is not compromised by the exemption and when another suitable means of verification of removal is employed. In these cases, the authenticated operative report must document the removal. Exceptions to sending specimens to the pathologist for evaluation could be made for such limited categories as foreign bodies, teeth, or other specimens that by their nature or condition do not permit fruitful examination.

Request the list of exemptions that have been approved by the governing body. Annotate on the survey report form if these exemptions appear inappropriate.

Select five medical records and annotate whether the exemptions contained therein are consistent with those exemptions previously approved.

Q-0029 §416.48 Condition for Coverage: Pharmaceutical Services

The ASC must provide drugs and biologicals in a safe and effective manner, in accordance with accepted professional practice, and under the direction of an individual designated responsible for pharmaceutical services.

Interpretive Guidelines §416.48

"Accepted professional practice" and "acceptable standards of practice" mean patient care standards established by national, state, and local professional associations regarding clinical use of drugs and biologicals.

There should be records of receipt and disposition of all controlled drugs.

The label of drug containers should have the name, strength, directions for use and expiration date of the drug.

Survey Procedures and Probes §416.48

Record whether there are procedures for disposal of discontinued, outdated, and deteriorated drugs. Drugs and biologicals must be current, not outdated, and properly refrigerated, if necessary. Annotate on the survey report form if no one is designated the responsibilities for pharmaceutical services.

Q-0030 §416.48(a) Standard: Administration of Drugs

Drugs must be administered according to established policies and acceptable standards of practice.

Q-0031 §416.48(a)

(1) Adverse reactions must be reported to the physician responsible for the patient and must be documented in the record.

Survey Procedures and Probes §416.48(a)(1)

The ASC must have policies and procedures in place covering the administration and preparation of drugs and reporting of adverse drug reactions. Request five patient records and note if the procedures are being followed.

Q-0032 §416.48(a)

(2) Blood and blood products must be administered only by physicians or registered nurses.

Survey Procedures and Probes §416.48(a)(2)

The ASC must have policies and procedures that identify who is authorized to administer blood and blood products.

Q-0033 §416.48(a)

(3) Orders given orally for drugs and biologicals must be followed by a written order and signed by the prescribing physician.

Survey Procedures and Probes §416.48(a)(3)

Record whether medication orders are signed by the physician.

Select five medication cards and annotate on the survey report form if they confirm the physician's order, i.e., that drug, dosage, and administration are as directed.

Q-0034 §416.49 Condition for Coverage: Laboratory and Radiology Services

If the ASC performs laboratory services, it must meet the requirements of part 493 of this chapter. If the ASC does not provide its own laboratory services, it must have procedures for obtaining routine and emergency laboratory services from a certified laboratory in accordance with part 493 of this chapter. The referral laboratory must be certified in the appropriate specialties and subspecialties of service to perform the referred tests in accordance with the requirements of part 493 of this chapter. The ASC must have procedures for obtaining radiology services, from a Medicare approved facility to meet the needs of patients.

Interpretive Guidelines §416.49

ASC policies and procedures should list the kinds of laboratory services that are provided directly by the facility, and services that are provided through a contractual agreement. Review the contractual agreements and determine if the referral laboratory is a CLIA-approved laboratory. Policies and procedures should encompass the following:

- A well-defined arrangement (need not be contractual) with outside services

- Laboratory services that are provided by the ASC

- Routine procedures for requesting lab tests and radiological exams

- Incorporate lab/radiological reports into patient records

When laboratory tests are performed prior to admission, the results should be readily available to the attending physician in the ASC.

If the facility provides directly for all radiological services, the surveyor is to apply either the Condition of Participation for Hospitals at §482.26 Radiology Department, or the Conditions for Coverage of portable x-ray services at §§405.1411-405.1416. If the services are provided for other than patients of the ASC, the facility could not be certified as an ASC.

When the ASC fails to meet either the radiology requirement for hospitals or portable x-ray requirement, then all radiology services must be obtained from a Medicare-approved facility. Note, however, that a Medicare-approved portable x-ray supplier is not a facility and cannot provide x-ray services to an ASC. Portable x-ray services must be furnished in a place of residence used as the patient's home (as detailed in 42 CFR 410.32(a)(2).

CMS proposed ASC Conditions of Participation

CMS proposed ASC Conditions of Participation

Health facilities, health professions, Medicare, reporting, and recordkeeping requirements.

For the reasons set forth in the preamble, the Centers for Medicare & Medicaid Services proposes to amend 42 CFR part 416 as follows:

PART 416—AMBULATORY SURGICAL SERVICES

1. The authority citation for part 416 continues to read as follows:

Authority: Secs. 1102 and 1871 of the Social Security Act (42 U.S.C. 1302 and 1395hh).

Subpart A—General Provisions and Definitions

2. Section Sec. 416.2 is amended by--

A. Revising the definition of "Ambulatory surgical center or ASC."

B. Adding the definition of "Overnight stay" in alphabetical order.

The revision and addition reads as follows:

Sec. 416.2 Definitions.

As used in this part:

> Ambulatory surgical center or ASC means any distinct entity that operates exclusively for the purpose of providing surgical services to patients not requiring an overnight stay following the surgical services, has an agreement with CMS to participate in Medicare as an ASC, and meets the conditions set forth in subparts B and C of this part.

* * * * *

> Overnight stay means the patient's recovery requires active monitoring by qualified medical personnel, regardless of whether it is provided in the ASC, beyond 11:59 p.m. of the day on which the surgical procedure was performed.

Subpart C--Specific Conditions for Coverage

3. Section 416.41 is revised to read as follows.

Sec. 416.41 Condition for coverage--Governing body and management.

The ASC must have a governing body that assumes full legal responsibility for determining, implementing, and monitoring policies governing the ASC's total operation; has oversight and accountability for the quality assurance and performance improvement program; and ensures that facility policies and programs are administered so as to provide quality health care in a safe environment, and creates and maintains a disaster preparedness plan.

A. Standard: Contract services. When services are provided through a contract with an outside resource, the ASC must assure that these services are provided in a safe and effective manner.

B. Standard: Hospitalization.

(1) The ASC must have an effective procedure for the immediate transfer, to a hospital, of patients requiring emergency medical care beyond the capabilities of the ASC.

(2) This hospital must be a local, Medicare-participating hospital or a local, nonparticipating hospital that meets the requirements for payment for emergency services under Sec. 482.2 of this chapter.

(3) The ASC must--

(i) Have a written transfer agreement with a hospital that meets the requirements of paragraph (b)(2) of this section; or

(ii) Ensure that all physicians performing surgery in the ASC have admitting privileges at a hospital that meets the requirements of paragraph (b)(2) of this section.

C. Standard: Disaster preparedness plan.

(1) The ASC must maintain a written disaster preparedness plan that provides for the emergency care of patients in the event of fire, natural disaster, functional failure of equipment, or other unexpected events or circumstances that are likely to threaten the health and safety of its patients.

(2) The ASC coordinates the plan with State and local agencies, as appropriate.

(3) The ASC conducts drills, at least annually, to test the plan's effectiveness. The ASC must complete a written evaluation of each drill and immediately implement any corrections to the plan.

4. Section 416.43 is revised to read as follows:

Sec. 416.43 Conditions for coverage--Quality assessment and performance improvement.

The ASC must develop, implement and maintain an ongoing, data-driven quality assessment and performance improvement (QAPI) program.

A. Standard: Program scope.

(1) The program must include, but not be limited to, an ongoing program that demonstrates measurable improvement in patient health outcomes, and improves patient safety by using quality indicators or performance measures associated with improved health outcomes and with the identification and reduction of medical errors.

(2) The ASC must measure, analyze, and track quality indicators, including adverse patient

events, infection control and other aspects of performance that includes processes of care and services furnished in the ASC.

B. Standard: Program data.

(1) The program must incorporate quality indicator data including patient care and other relevant data regarding services furnished in the ASC into its QAPI program.

(2) The ASC must use the data collected to--

(i) Monitor the effectiveness and safety of its services, and quality of its care.

(ii) Identify opportunities that could lead to improvements and changes in its patient care.

C. Standard: Program activities.

(1) The ASC must set priorities for its performance improvement activities that--

(i) Focus on high risk, high volume and problem-prone areas.

(ii) Consider incidence, prevalence and severity of problems in those areas.

(iii) Affect health outcomes, patient safety and quality of care.

(2) Performance improvement activities must track adverse patient events, examine their causes, implement improvements and ensure that improvements are sustained over time.

(3) The ASC must implement preventive strategies throughout the facility targeting adverse patient events and ensure that all staff are familiar with these strategies.

D. Standard: Performance improvement projects.

[[Page 50486]]

(1) The number and scope of distinct improvement projects conducted annually must reflect the scope and complexity of the ASC's services and operations.

(2) The ASC must document the projects that are being conducted.

The documentation at a minimum must include the reason(s) for implementing the project, and a description of the project's results.

E. Standard: Governing body responsibilities. The governing body must ensure that the QAPI--

(1) Program is defined, implemented and maintained by the ASC.

(2) Program addresses the ASC's priorities and that all improvements are evaluated for effectiveness.

(3) Data collection methods, frequency and details are appropriate.

(4) Program expectations for safety are clearly established.

(5) Resources are adequately allocated for implementing the facility's program.

5. Section 416.49 is revised to read as follows:

Sec. 416.49 Condition for coverage--Laboratory and radiologic services.

A. Standard: Laboratory. If the ASC performs laboratory services, it must meet the requirements of part 493 of this chapter. If the ASC does not provide its own laboratory services, it must have procedures for obtaining routine and emergency laboratory services from a certified laboratory in accordance with part 493 of this chapter. The referral laboratory must be certified in the appropriate specialties and subspecialties of service to perform the referred tests in accordance with the requirements of part 493 of this chapter.

B. Standard: Radiologic services.

(1) The ASC must have procedures for obtaining radiological services from a Medicare approved facility to meet the needs of patients.

(2) When radiologic services are medically necessary and integral to the performance of surgical procedures the ASC must meet the requirements of the Conditions for Coverage for Portable X-ray Services under Sec. 486.100 through Sec. 486.110 of this chapter if it is furnishing these services directly. Radiologic services furnished under arrangement must be performed by an entity that is certified by Medicare as a supplier of portable x-ray services by meeting the Conditions for Coverage for Portable X-ray Services.

6. Add new Sec. 416.50 to read as follows:

Sec. 416.50 Condition for coverage--Patients' rights.

The ASC must inform the patient or the patient's representative of the patient's rights, and must protect and promote the exercise of such rights.

    A. Standard: Notice of rights.

      (1) The ASC must provide the patient or the patient's representative with verbal and written notice of the patient's rights prior to furnishing care to the patient and in a language and manner that the patient or patient representative understands. In addition, the ASC must--

        (i) Post the written notice of patient rights in a place or places within the ASC likely to be noticed by patients (or their representative, if applicable) waiting for treatment. Notice of rights must include the name, address, and telephone number for a representative in the State agency to whom patients can report complaints about ASCs, as well as the Web site for the Medicare Beneficiary Ombudsman.

        (ii) Disclose, if applicable, physician financial interests or ownership in the ASC facility in accordance with part 420 of this subchapter. Disclosure information must be in writing and furnished to the patient prior to the first visit to the ASC.

      (2) Advance directives. The ASC must comply with the following requirements:

        (i) Provide the patient or representative with verbal and written information concerning its policies on advance directives, including a description of applicable State law and, if requested, official State advance directive forms.

        (ii) Inform the patient or representative of the patient's right to make informed decisions regarding their care.

        (iii) Document in a prominent part of the patient's current medical record, whether or not the individual has executed an advance directive.

      (3) Submission and investigation of grievances.

        (i) The ASC must establish clearly explained procedures for documenting the existence, submission, investigation and disposition of a patient's written or verbal grievance to the ASC.

        (ii) All alleged violations/grievances relating, but not limited to, mistreatment, neglect, verbal, mental, sexual or physical abuse, must be fully documented.

        (iii) All allegations must be immediately reported to a person in authority in the ASC, the State and local bodies having jurisdiction, and the State survey agency if warranted.

(iv) The grievance process must specify time frames for review of the grievance and the provision of a response.

(v) The ASC, in responding to the grievance, must investigate all grievances made by a patient or the patient's representative regarding treatment or care that is (or fails to be) furnished.

(vi) The ASC must document how the grievance was addressed, as well as provide the patient with written notice of its decision. The decision must contain the name of an ASC contact person, the steps taken to investigate the grievance, the results of the grievance process, and the date the grievance process was completed.

B. Standard: Exercise of rights and respect for property and person.

(1) The patient has the right to--

(i) Exercise his or her rights without being subjected to discrimination or reprisal.

(ii) Voice grievances regarding treatment or care that is (or fails to be) furnished.

(iii) Be fully informed about a treatment or procedure and the expected outcome before it is performed.

(2) If a patient is adjudged incompetent under State law by a court of proper jurisdiction, the rights of the patient are exercised by the person appointed under State law to act on the patient's behalf.

(3) If a State court has not adjudged a patient incompetent, any legal representative designated by the patient in accordance with State law may exercise the patient's rights to the extent allowed by State law.

C. Standard: Privacy and safety. The patient has the right to--

(1) Personal privacy.

(2) Receive care in a safe setting.

(3) Be free from all forms of abuse or harassment.

D. Standard: Confidentiality of clinical records. The patient has the right to confidentiality of his or her clinical records maintained by the ASC. Access to or release of patient information and clinical records is permitted only with written consent of the patient or the patient's representative or as authorized by law.

7. Add new Sec. 416.51 to read as follows:

Sec. 416.51 Conditions for coverage--Infection Control.

The Ambulatory Surgical Center (ASC) must maintain an infection control program for patients and ASC staff that seeks to minimize infections and communicable diseases.

A. Standard: Sanitary environment. The ASC must provide a functional and sanitary environment for the provision of surgical services by adhering to professionally acceptable standards of practice.

[[Page 50487]]

B. Standard: Infection control program. The ASC must maintain an ongoing program designed to prevent, control, and investigate infections and communicable diseases. The program is-- (1) Under the direction of a designated and qualified professional who has training in infection control.

(2) An integral part of the ASC's quality assessment and performance improvement program; and

(3) Responsible for providing a plan of action for preventing, identifying and managing infections and communicable diseases and for immediately implementing corrective and preventive measures that result in improvement.

8. Add new Sec. 416.52 to read as follows:

Sec. 416.52 Conditions for coverage--Patient admission, assessment and discharge.

The ASC must develop specific assessments for each patient's medical needs with respect to their visit to the ASC.

A. Standard: Admission and pre-surgical assessment.

(1) Not more than 30 days before the date of the scheduled surgery, each patient must have a comprehensive medical history and physical assessment completed by a physician (as defined in section 1861(r) of the Act) or other qualified practitioner in accordance with State law and ASC policy.

(2) Upon admission, each patient must have a pre-surgical assessment that includes, at a minimum, an updated medical record entry documenting an examination for any changes in

the patient's condition since the most recently documented medical history and physical assessment. The assessment must include documentation to determine the patient's physical and mental ability to undergo the surgical procedure, and any allergies to drugs and biologicals.

(3) The patient's medical history and physical assessment must be placed in the patient's medical record before the surgical procedure is started.

B. Standard: Post-surgical assessment.

(1) A thorough assessment of the patient's post-surgical condition must be completed and documented in the medical record.

(2) Post-surgical needs must be addressed and included in the discharge notes.

C. Standard: Discharge. The ASC must--

(1) Provide each patient with written discharge instructions.

(2) Ensure the patient has a safe transition to home and that the post-surgical needs are met.

(3) Ensure each patient has a discharge order, signed by a physician or the qualified practitioner who performed the surgery or procedure unless otherwise specified by State law. The discharge order must indicate that the patient has been evaluated for proper anesthesia and medical recovery.

Authority: (Catalog of Federal Domestic Assistance Program No. 93.778, Medical Assistance Program).

(Catalog of Federal Domestic Assistance Program No. 93.773, Medicare--Hospital Insurance; and Program No. 93.774, Medicare--Supplementary Medical Insurance Program)

Dated: January 30, 2007.

Leslie V. Norwalk,

Acting Administrator, Centers for Medicare & Medicaid Services.

 Approved: May 22, 2007.

Michael O. Leavitt,

Secretary.

Editorial Note: This document was received at the Office of the Federal Register on August 21, 2007.

[FR Doc. 07-4148 Filed 8-24-07; 4:00 pm]

BILLING CODE 4120-01-P